100 Questions & Answers About Lymphoma
Third Edition

Peter Holman, MD
Moores Cancer Center
University of California, San Diego, CA

Gregory Bociek, MD
Associate Professor
Internal Medicine Division of Hematology
University of Nebraska Medical Center
Oncology/Hematology Division
Omaha, NE

Jodi Garrett, RN
Moores Cancer Center
University of California, San Diego, CA

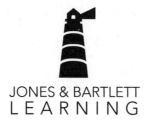

JONES & BARTLETT
LEARNING

World Headquarters
Jones & Bartlett Learning
5 Wall Street
Burlington, MA 01803
978-443-5000
info@jblearning.com
www.jblearning.com

Jones & Bartlett Learning books and products are available through most bookstores and online booksellers.
To contact Jones & Bartlett Learning directly, call 800-832-0034, fax 978-443-8000, or visit our website, www.jblearning.com.

Production Credits

Executive Acquisitions Editor: Nancy Anastasi Duffy
Production Assistant: Alex Schab
Marketing Manager: Jennifer Sharp
Manufacturing and Inventory Control Supervisor: Amy Bacus
Composition: Miranda Design Studio, Inc.
Cover Design: Kristin E. Parker
Rights and Photo Research Coordinator: Ashley Dos Santos
Cover Image: Top: © PhotoDisc, Bottom Right: © PhotoDisc, Bottom Left: © PhotoDisc
Printing and Binding: Edwards Brothers Malloy
Cover Printing: Edwards Brothers Malloy

Library of Congress Cataloging-in-Publication Data
Holman, Peter, M.D.
   100 questions and answers about lymphoma / Peter Holman, Gregory Bociek, Jodi Garrett. — Third edition.
      pages cm
   ISBN 978-1-284-02256-8
   1. Lymphomas—Popular works. 2. Lymphomas—Miscellanea. I. Bociek, Gregory. II. Garrett, Jodi. III. Title.
   IV. Title: One hundred questions and answers about lymphoma.
   RC280.L9H65 2015
   616.99ʹ446—dc23
                                        2014021067
6048

Printed in the United States of America
18 17 16 15 14   10 9 8 7 6 5 4 3 2 1

According to the American Cancer Society, approximately 79,000 new cases of lymphoma will be diagnosed in the United States in 2014. Of these, approximately 70,000 cases will be non-Hodgkin lymphomas, and the remaining cases (9,000) will be Hodgkin lymphomas. Since the early 1970s, for unclear reasons, the incidence of lymphoma has doubled and continues to rise.

The term "lymphoma" actually describes many different but related diseases. Although there is overlap, the different lymphomas tend to affect people in different ways. There are even some types of lymphoma that may not always require treatment; for most lymphomas, however, there are a number of treatment choices that can be made in any particular situation. It is therefore a major challenge for individuals receiving such a diagnosis to obtain the relevant information necessary to be an active participant in their care. The Internet is a very useful source of information, but it also contains much disinformation that can be more damaging and frightening than helpful.

In this book, written for patients and their caregivers, we (two physicians and a nurse) have attempted to provide an understanding of lymphoma—both non-Hodgkin lymphoma and Hodgkin lymphoma—that will assist you in understanding this disease and coping with the daily pressures of the fight against lymphoma. In addition, the Appendix includes links to sites with additional information about lymphoma-related clinical research and clinical trials. We hope you find it useful.

PART ONE

The Basics: Understanding the Immune and Circulatory Systems

What is the immune system?

How do the components of the immune system function?

What is bone marrow?

More . . .

1. What is the immune system?

Lymphoma

Cancer of the lymphocytes.

Immune system

The complex system by which the body protects itself from harmful outside invaders.

Bacteria

One class of infectious agents.

Viruses

Tiny infectious agents that require other cells for their growth and survival.

Lymphatic channels

The tiny vessels that connect the lymph glands.

Lymph nodes

Another term for lymph glands.

Lymph glands

The large collections of lymphocytes that exist at intervals throughout the lymph system. They can get big and painful in response to an infection.

Tonsils

Large lymph nodes present in the back of the throat.

All types of **lymphoma** arise from cells that are part of the normal **immune system**. Understanding the immune system is therefore important to understanding lymphoma. Your immune system is what protects you from illnesses by recognizing and eliminating dangerous foreign (abnormal) substances. This system is your main defense against all infections (illness arising from invasion from outside organisms, such as **bacteria** or **viruses**) and also plays an important role in how your body responds to many diseases, including lymphoma and other cancers. Individuals in whom the immune system is not functioning properly have an increased risk of certain cancers (including lymphoma), infections, and autoimmune disorders, which are illnesses characterized by organ damage as a result of self-recognition by cells of the immune system.

The immune system consists of a variety of important components, including a meshwork-like circulation system of **lymphatic channels** throughout the body that connects the **lymph nodes** or **lymph glands**, the **tonsils**, the **spleen**, and the **thymus** (**Figure 1**). The lymphatic channels run alongside the blood circulation and connect with the **bone marrow**. The spleen is an organ that is normally the size of your fist and can become enlarged when affected by lymphoma or other disorders. It essentially functions like a very large lymph node and is located in the upper left part of the abdomen, beside the stomach. The thymus is another lymphoid organ that is located behind the breastbone (sternum) in children and young adults; it becomes relatively inactive in older adults. The circulating **lymph fluid** contains large numbers of **lymphocytes—white blood cells** that fight disease. The lymphocytes are the "foot soldiers" of the immune system, directly responsible for destroying invading organisms or abnormal cells.

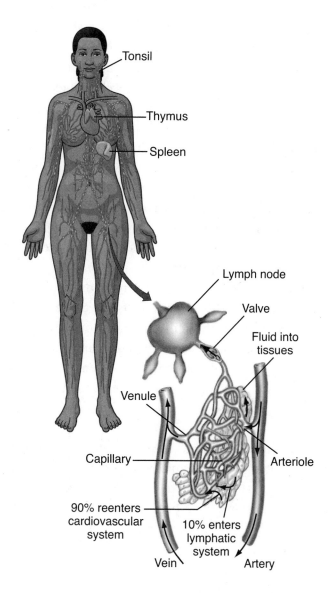

Figure 1 The lymphatic system consists of the lymphatic vessels and ducts, lymph nodes (which are distributed throughout the body), tonsils, thymus gland, and spleen. The enlarged diagram of a lymph node and vessels shows the path of the excess fluid that leaves the arteriole end of a capillary bed, enters the adjacent tissue spaces, and is absorbed by lymphatic capillaries.

Reprinted from Alters, *Biology: Understanding Life*, Fourth Ed. Copyright © 2000 Jones and Bartlett Publishers, LLC.

Spleen

The large lymph node-like organ under the lower left ribs.

Thymus

An organ behind the breastbone that is important for the development of an immune response, especially in children.

Bone marrow

Soft substance inside many bones in the body where the blood cells are produced.

Lymph fluid

The fluid that carries lymphocytes around the body.

Lymphocytes

The main type of cell that makes up the immune system. It is the abnormal cell in lymphoma.

White blood cells

Blood cells that are most important for fighting infection.

3

B cell

A type of lymphocyte.

T cell

One of the major types of lymphocytes.

Tissues

A collection of cells of a similar type with a similar function.

Autoimmune disease

An illness in which a person's own immune system mistakenly begins to see certain parts of its own body as foreign, resulting in immunologically driven inflammatory damage to the tissues affected.

Rheumatoid arthritis

An autoimmune disorder associated with destruction and deformity of joints.

Systemic lupus erythematosus

A disease in which the immune system attacks the body, causing inflammatory damage to multiple organs, including the skin, kidneys, heart, or brain.

The two main types of lymphocytes (**B cells** and **T cells**) act together with other immune cells to mount an attack in response to foreign invaders such as infections. The manner in which disease cells are recognized is essential in the body's success or failure in fending off an illness. For example, under certain circumstances, lymphocytes mistake an individual's own body **tissues** for foreign substances. In such cases, this error results in an immune attack on normal tissues; such attacks are called **autoimmune diseases** and include illnesses such as **rheumatoid arthritis** and **systemic lupus erythematosus**. It is important to note that in most cancers, including lymphoma, the immune system fails in the opposite way—it does not recognize the cancer cells as foreign and therefore allows the cancer to grow unchecked. Clearly, the ability of the immune system to respond appropriately is one key factor in cancer treatment, and failure of the immune system to eradicate abnormal cells may result in the development of cancers including lymphoma.

The body initially "trains" its own T cells to distinguish foreign proteins from normal body proteins. This training occurs in the thymus during childhood, when the thymus is still an active organ; after adolescence, the thymus shrinks (or involutes) and has little or no function in adults.

2. How do the components of the immune system function?

Two circulatory systems transport immune cells around the body. The blood circulatory system carries blood from the heart to the lungs, where **red blood cells** receive oxygen, and then onward via the **arteries** throughout the body where oxygen and nutrients are delivered to tissues, allowing normal metabolism to occur. At the same time, carbon dioxide, waste, and toxic matter are transported to the lungs, liver, or kidneys for elimination from the body. In addition to this function of supplying oxygen and removing waste substances, the blood also carries the disease- and injury-fighting white blood cells, which include the lymphocytes and a number of other cells (described in Questions 4 and 5 on pages 8 and 9), as well as many other types of protein, including those that are important for blood clotting.

The lesser-known circulatory system is the lymphatic system, which works alongside the blood circulatory system in fighting disease. The lymphatic circulation transports the lymph fluid—rich in lymphocytes— around the body in lymph channels in much the same way as blood is transported via arteries and **veins**. Lymphocytes are produced in the bone marrow (see Question 3 on page 7), after which they travel through both the bloodstream and lymphatic channels to the lymph nodes and/or the thymus (in children and adolescents) and then back into the bloodstream. The lymphatic channels that compose the lymphatic circulatory system consist of tiny, thin, leaky vessels that carry lymph fluid back toward the heart. They usually run alongside the veins, which likewise carry blood back to the heart from various parts of the body.

At frequent intervals along the lymphatic channels, large clusters of lymphocytes occur. These are the lymph nodes or glands in which lymphocytes often first encounter a foreign protein or **antigen**. When a lymphocyte recognizes a protein as foreign, it sends out signals to other lymphocytes, recruiting help in mounting an immune response directed at ridding the body of the foreign

Red blood cells

The most common type of blood cells that carry oxygen around the body. They carry oxygen to the tissues of the body and help eliminate carbon dioxide from the body by carrying it back to the lungs for elimination.

Arteries

The vessels that carry blood cells containing oxygen to the organs and tissues of the body.

Veins

Blood vessels that return blood to the heart.

Antigen

Any substance that can induce an immune response. Antigens include infections or cancer cells.

THE BASICS: UNDERSTANDING THE IMMUNE AND CIRCULATORY SYSTEMS protein. Lymphocytes and other inflammatory cells accumulate in the region, and when activated through their encounter with the foreign substance, they secrete chemical messengers that orchestrate the appropriate immune response. An example of this is the development of red, swollen tonsils (which are large lymphatic organs in the throat) during an infection or a cold. Similarly, lymph nodes in other sites can become enlarged and painful during a serious infection. This accumulation reflects the immune system's attempt to control and eliminate the infection. Lymph nodes are located throughout the body, but, when enlarged, they are most easily felt in the neck, armpits, and groin. Collections of nodes also occur in the chest, between the lungs, and in the abdomen, where they are found alongside the **aorta** and the **inferior vena cava**, the major blood vessel, which carries blood away from and back to the heart.

The spleen is a specialized organ within the immune system and functions in many respects as a very large lymph node. The spleen is essentially a very large collection of lymphocytes and is another site where lymphocytes can come into contact with foreign proteins. Certain infections, including **infectious mononucleosis** (commonly called glandular fever) and **malaria**, can result in an enlarged spleen. When this occurs, your physician may feel the spleen when examining your abdomen. Since a normal sized spleen cannot be felt, the ability to feel a spleen on an examination implies something abnormal that requires further explanation. Under certain circumstances, the spleen may need to be surgically removed. If this is necessary, especially in children, antibiotics may be prescribed to prevent certain types of infection. Although you can live a normal life without a spleen, it is an important part of the immune system, providing significant protection against some types of

Aorta

The main blood vessel (artery) that carries blood from the heart to the smaller arteries, thereby delivering blood to all parts of the body.

Inferior vena cava

The large vein that carries blood back toward the heart.

Infectious mononucleosis

A viral infection caused by the Epstein-Barr virus. Also called glandular fever.

Malaria

An infection caused by a parasite that is transmitted by mosquitoes.

infection; thus, patients without a spleen should seek medical attention quickly in the event of an infection.

You can think of these components as a combined defensive army that is fighting a continuing battle against would-be invaders. The lymphocyte "ground troops" are born and "armed" within the bone marrow (during childhood, they are also sent out for "training" in the thymus). Then they patrol the body via the lymphatic system and battle invaders in the nodes and, during cases of very serious invasion, in the tonsils and spleen as well.

3. What is bone marrow?

The bone marrow is a soft spongy substance that is present inside many of the bones in your body. It is where all blood cells are produced from the blood-forming **stem cells**, responsible for the production of red blood cells, white blood cells, and **platelets**. All of these cells go through a number of different stages of maturation within the bone marrow before mature cells are released into the bloodstream. If the bloodstream becomes deficient in any type of cell, such as a low red blood cell count in a patient with **anemia**, the bone marrow may attempt to replace the missing red blood cells by increasing production. In adults, functional bone marrow is present in the skull, backbones (vertebrae), ribs, hips, and pelvic bones and at the top ends of the **humerus** (upper arm bone) and **femur** (thigh bone). Normally, fat cells take up approximately half the bone marrow space; the other half consists of the blood-forming cells. An increased proportion of cells to fat as seen under a microscope can be a pathologist's first sign of an abnormality in the marrow. The bone marrow can be involved in many types of lymphoma, explaining the need for bone marrow examinations.

Stem cells

A type of cell that can produce red cells, white cells, and platelets.

Platelets

Tiny blood cells that are produced in the bone marrow and are important for blood clotting.

Anemia

A condition marked by a low hemoglobin level.

Humerus

The major bone connecting the shoulder to the elbow.

Femur

The thigh bone.

4. What are lymphocytes and natural killer (NK) cells?

Lymphocytes are one type of white blood cell (other white blood cells are described in Question 5 on page 9; see **Figure 2**). Although they fight disease, lymphocytes are the "foot soldiers" of the immune system, and it is specifically these cells that lymphoma affects (see Question 1 on page 2). The two main types of lymphocytes, B and T cells, have different roles in working to eliminate foreign proteins (antigens) from the body, but they work together to achieve the same result of preventing and eliminating illnesses. A third type of lymphocyte is the NK cell, which accounts for about 10% of lymphocytes. NK cells and T cells share common precursor cells and have many similarities.

B-lymphocytes (or B cells) are historically named for where they come from in chicken embryos, an organ called the "bursa of Fabricius," although humans have no such organ. Both B and T lymphocytes are produced in our bone marrow. T lymphocytes (or T cells) are so called because of the important role that the thymus plays in their development.

From the bone marrow, T cells circulate throughout the body using both blood vessels and lymphatic channels. T and B cells look identical when blood is examined under a microscope, but the types of molecules or protein substances on their surfaces can help to distinguish them. Specialized laboratory equipment found in most hospitals or clinical laboratories can be used to distinguish the different types of lymphocytes on the basis of these proteins. It is the growth and accumulation of large numbers of abnormal lymphocytes that results in the lymph node enlargement that occurs in lymphoma.

NK cells account for most of the large granular lymphocytes present in the blood. Abnormalities result in a number of types of rare, unusual lymphoma or leukemia. NK cells play an important role in the function of the immune system. Individuals born without NK cells experience recurrent severe viral infections.

5. What are the other types of blood cells?

In addition to lymphocytes, the bone marrow produces many other types of blood cells (**Figure 2**) that are the offspring of a very important bone marrow cell called the **hematopoietic stem cell**, which can produce all of the blood cells ("hematopoietic" is derived from the Greek words *haimatos*, which means blood, and *poiein*, which means to make). Embryonic stem cells, the subject of much ongoing scientific, ethical, and political discussion, differ from these cells, as they can give rise to cells of many more different tissues than the hematopoietic stem cell. Thus, when stem cells are discussed in this context, we mean strictly the hematopoietic stem cells that give rise to blood cells.

Hematopoietic stem cell

The most immature cell that has the capacity to develop into/generate red cells, white blood cells, and platelets throughout a person's life.

The main groups of blood cells are red cells, white cells, and platelets. As mentioned previously, the B and T lymphocytes are only two of a number of different types of white blood cells.

White Blood Cells

All of the white cells are produced in the bone marrow. From there, they make their way into the bloodstream, where they circulate for varying lengths of time before moving into the tissues of the body. They can carry out their functions in the bloodstream or various tissues.

	BLOOD CELL TYPE	DESCRIPTION	FUNCTION	LIFE SPAN
RED BLOOD CELLS	Erythrocyte	Flat disk with a central depression, no nucleus, contain hemoglobin.	Transport oxygen (O_2) and carbon dioxide (CO_2).	About 120 days.
WHITE BLOOD CELLS (LEUKOCYTES) — Granulocytes	Neutrophil	Spherical; with many-lobed nucleus, no hemoglobin, pink-purple **cytoplasmic granules**.	Cellular defense-phagocytosis of small microorganisms.	Hours to 3 days.
	Eosinophil	Spherical; two-lobed nucleus, no hemoglobin, orange-red staining **cytoplasmic granules**.	Cellular defense—phagocytosis of large microorganisms such as parasitic worms, releases anti-inflammatory substances in allergic reactions.	8 to 12 days.
	Basophil	Spherical; generally two-lobed nucleus, no hemoglobin large purple staining **cytoplasmic granules**.	Inflammatory response—contain granules that rupture and release chemicals enhancing inflammatory response.	Hours to 3 days.
WHITE BLOOD CELLS (LEUKOCYTES) — Agranulocytes	Monocyte	Spherical; **single nucleus** shaped like kidney bean, no cytoplasmic granules, cytoplasm often blue in color.	Converted to macrophages, which are large cells that entrap microorganisms and other foreign matter.	Days to months.
	B lymphocyte	Spherical; round **singular nucleus**, no cytoplasmic granules.	Immune system response and regulation, antibody production sometimes causes allergic response.	Days to years.
	T lymphocyte	Spherical; round **singular nucleus**, no cytoplasmic granules.	Immune system response and regulation; cellular immune response.	Days to years.
PLATELETS	Platelets	Irregularly shaped fragments, very small pink staining granules.	Control blood clotting or coagulation.	7 to 10 days.

Figure 2 Types of blood cells.

Neutrophil

The main type of white blood cell. It is especially important for fighting bacterial infections.

Nucleus

The central part of the cell. It contains the genetic information for that cell.

Cytoplasm

The fluid part of a cell that surrounds the central nucleus.

Neutrophils, a particularly important cell in defense against bacterial infections, are the most common type of white blood cell. Lymphocytes are the second most frequent white blood cell. Neutrophils are easily identified under a microscope with a **nucleus** that is divided up into three or four lobes. The **cytoplasm** (the part of the cell that surrounds the nucleus) of the neutrophils contains **granules**, which in turn contain chemicals (**enzymes**) that are important for killing bacteria. When someone has a bacterial infection, the number of white cells in the blood normally increases, mostly because of an increase in neutrophils.

Chemotherapy, which is a name for certain types of medications used to treat disease—cancer, in this case—can be used to kill the cancer cells, but it also prevents the bone marrow's production of neutrophils. In general, cells that multiply rapidly (i.e., have a higher proliferation rate) are more sensitive to the effects of chemotherapy. Neutrophils have a high proliferation rate, and, as such people receiving chemotherapy have periods when low neutrophil counts occur, placing them at an increased risk of bacterial infection. For this reason, many patients on chemotherapy also receive **growth factors**, which help increase the neutrophil count and shorten the period of time that the neutrophils are low. In certain circumstances, patients may also be prescribed antibiotics in an attempt to prevent infections.

Other white blood cells include **monocytes, eosinophils**, and basophils. The monocytes are also important in preventing and controlling bacterial infections. Eosinophils are important in responding to parasites and have a role in allergic reactions. The white blood cell count is usually normal in people when they are diagnosed with lymphoma, but some types of lymphoma can first be identified by finding an elevated white blood cell count. It is important to know which types of white blood cells are present in the blood, as even when the total white blood cell count is normal, lymphoma cells can be found circulating in the blood. When tested in a clinical laboratory, the white blood cell count is reported as an absolute number, and a differential count is usually given, identifying the relative percentage of neutrophils, lymphocytes, eosinophils, and basophils. The absolute number of the different white blood cells can then be calculated.

Granules

Small particles inside white blood cells that contain enzymes.

Enzymes

Chemical messengers within the body.

Chemotherapy

Drugs used to treat a disease; the different types of drugs used to treat cancer.

Growth factors

Chemicals that can be injected to stimulate the production of blood cells.

Monocytes

One type of white blood cell.

Eosinophils

One type of white blood cell.

THE BASICS: UNDERSTANDING THE IMMUNE AND CIRCULATORY SYSTEMS

Red Blood Cells

Red blood cells, the most common type of blood cells, do not have a nucleus but contain a red pigment called **hemoglobin**, which is essential to life because it allows oxygen to be carried around the body. The presence of a low hemoglobin level is referred to as anemia and is easily discovered by performing a **complete blood count** (**CBC**). The most common reasons for people with lymphoma to develop anemia are the presence of lymphoma in the bone marrow or the effects of chemotherapy on the bone marrow.

Platelets

Platelets are another identifiable component of blood. They are fragments produced in the bone marrow from very large cells in the bone marrow called **megakaryocytes**. Platelets are very important in preventing and stopping bleeding and bruising. Both the presence of lymphoma in the bone marrow and the effects of chemotherapy on the marrow can affect the production of platelets. Rarely, low platelet counts can result from the production of auto-antibodies that bind to platelets. These antibody-coated platelets then get removed from the circulation by the spleen. Signs of a low platelet count include easy or spontaneous bruising, nose bleeding (epistaxis), or menstrual periods that are heavier and/or longer than normal (menorrhagia). Platelet transfusions may be warranted to reduce the risk of bleeding or to stop bleeding under certain circumstances.

The platelet count can also sometimes be high in patients with lymphoma or other cancers, as the body may react to the presence of cancer, infection, or some types of inflammation by releasing chemicals or **cytokines** that stimulate megakaryocytes to make more platelets. With treatment, the platelet count will generally return to normal.

Hemoglobin

A protein present in red blood cells that carries oxygen.

Complete blood count (CBC)

A blood test that takes looks at the red cell count, the hemoglobin, the white count, and the platelet count.

Megakaryocytes

The bone marrow cells that produce platelets.

Cytokines

Chemicals produced by T lymphocytes in order to generate an immune response.

6. How does the immune system fight infection?

The immune system has two main overlapping strategies to defend against foreign proteins. One approach uses the **humoral immune response**, and the foot soldiers for this mode of attack are the B cells. The other approach is the **cellular immune response**, which employs predominantly T cells. The two strategies generally act in concert to eliminate a foreign substance.

The humoral immune response uses **antibodies** to eliminate foreign protein. Antibodies are Y-shaped proteins. Each arm can attach to the foreign protein in much the same way as a key fits in a lock. The arms of the Y bind to the foreign protein, and the leg attaches to another type of immune cell called a **phagocyte**, which then removes the foreign protein coated with antibody from the circulation. **Monoclonal antibodies** used in the treatment of lymphoma and other cancers are designed to interact with target proteins on the surface of lymphoma cells or other cancer cells, and at least part of their ability to kill cancer cells is based on the antibody-coated cancer cell interacting with other cells in the normal immune system.

When specific B cells interact with and recognize a substance as foreign, they receive signals to develop into antibody-secreting cells. These cells are called **plasma cells**, which are found mostly in the spleen but are also common in the bone marrow. Normally, there is one pool of B cells for each different foreign protein that anybody might encounter over the course of a lifetime. When exposed to that foreign protein, the specific pool of B cells that can react to that foreign protein is stimulated to develop into plasma cells. The resulting population of plasma cells produces a specific antibody that

Humoral immune response

An immune response that uses antibodies rather than cells to destroy an antigen (foreign protein).

Cellular immune response

The part of the immune response that uses lymphocytes to directly remove antigens. In contrast, the humoral immune response uses antibodies to remove antigens.

Antibodies

Specialized proteins of the immune system that help fight infections. They can also be created to recognize proteins on cancer cells, as in some types of lymphoma treatments.

Phagocyte

A cell that scavenges other cells.

Monoclonal antibodies

Antibodies that bind to a specific target on the surface of lymphoma or other cancer cells.

is capable of attaching itself to the foreign protein. The attachment of the antibody to the foreign protein marks that protein for removal from the circulation.

Some of the B cells that recognize a foreign substance do not become plasma cells, but instead act to recruit T cells to help fight the foreign invader. The type of immune response that results from T-cell involvement is called the cellular immune response. This component of the immune system does not use antibodies but rather T cells. When T cells are activated by an encounter with a foreign protein, they generate chemicals called **lymphokines**. These in turn activate an entire host of immune cells including phagocytes, with the end result being the elimination of the infection. Lymphokines and similar substances called cytokines are responsible for many of the symptoms such as fever and aches that occur during viral infections such as the flu.

7. How is the immune system important in lymphoma?

The immune system is designed to recognize foreign proteins, and the way it does this is most evident in the responses seen with infection. However, the immune system also plays a role in surveying the body for abnormal cells that, if not removed, can become cancerous. All cancers are in some way the result of an imbalance between the normal rate of cell growth and/or the normal rate of programmed cell death in a particular tissue or organ. All cancers start out as an abnormality that occurs in a single cell. This abnormal cell develops a feature that somehow allows it to grow abnormally or survive better than its normal counterparts—that is, it develops a survival advantage. In order to recognize an abnormal cell as foreign, the cells of the immune system need to recognize a protein on the surface of the cell as abnormal. In lymphoma and many other cancers, the proteins on the surface of the lymphoma cell still appear normal since they started out as normal cells before they became malignant. This explains to a large extent why the patient's own immune response against a particular cancer is generally weak or absent.

All lymphomas arise from abnormalities in cells of the immune system, specifically the lymphocytes. In some cases, the lymphoma may occur as a result of some lymphocytes overreacting to certain types of infections. It is widely thought that many tissues develop small numbers of abnormal cells that have the potential to develop into cancers, but the immune system's recognition of these cells results in their safe removal. Therefore, a failure of the immune system to recognize the abnormal cells before they become a cancer is one mechanism whereby cancers, including lymphoma, can presumably occur.

It therefore appears that strategies designed to improve immune function or the immune system's recognition of abnormal cells could be a useful and unique way to treat cancers. Approximately a decade ago a number of investigators began laboratory-based experiments and subsequently clinical trials focusing on ways to make cancer cells more recognizable to the immune system. Cancer **vaccines** were designed with this goal in mind, but to date such **clinical trials** have failed to demonstrate a consistent clinical benefit to this particular strategy.

In some types of lymphoma, such as **indolent lymphomas**, the cells grow very slowly and patients may not require therapy for months to years after diagnosis. During that time the lymph node enlargement can

Vaccine

An injection given to stimulate an immune response.

Clinical trials

Research studies evaluating promising new treatments in patients.

Indolent lymphomas

A group of lymphomas that are generally slow growing and are usually treated only if causing important symptoms or signs of organ damage.

wax and wane (i.e., appear larger at times and smaller at other times). This is felt to reflect the immune system's attempt to control the lymphoma. This observation suggests that ways to enhance the immune system may allow for improved control of these types of lymphoma and possibly even a cure.

The treatment of lymphoma itself can have a significant impact on the immune system. The presence of lymphoma can impair the ability of the immune system to respond to infection, and this can be improved with treatment by controlling the lymphoma; however, the treatment of the lymphoma itself can further impair the functioning of the immune system.

PART TWO

Diagnosis and Classification of Lymphoma

What is lymphoma?

What is the difference between Hodgkin lymphoma and non-Hodgkin lymphoma?

What are the symptoms of lymphoma?

More . . .

8. What is lymphoma?

Lymphoma is cancer of the immune/lymphatic system, specifically the lymphocytes, in which an abnormality occurs in one lymphocyte that provides the cell with a growth or survival advantage, allowing the cell to divide and grow abnormally, or live longer than it usually would. Like all cancer cells, the abnormal lymphocyte does not obey the signals that control normal cell behavior. This allows more of the abnormal cells to grow or survive, eventually developing into a large collection of abnormal lymphocytes, which, when big enough to be detected by a physical examination or an X-ray, is called a tumor or mass. A **biopsy** can then be performed, allowing a **pathologist** to diagnose a lymphoma if one is present.

Most commonly, the abnormal growth of lymphocytes occurs in the lymph nodes, which then become enlarged. Abnormal lymphocytes can also collect in the bone marrow, blood, spleen, or other sites such as the **gastrointestinal tract**, lungs, or brain. In certain types of lymphoma, it is common or characteristic for the skin to be involved.

Lymphoma is actually a very broad term that applies to many different disorders that all have many features in common. Lymphomas all arise from an abnormality occurring in a single lymphocyte. There are many different types of lymphocytes, and the cancer-causing abnormality that occurs in the cell can occur at any point in the "life cycle" of the lymphocyte. As a result, there are many different types of lymphomas that can develop, making the classification of lymphomas very complicated.

Lymphoma

Cancer of the lymphatic system, specifically the lymphocytes, in which an abnormality occurs in one lymphocyte that provides the cell with a growth advantage, allowing the cell to divide and grow abnormally

Biopsy

The removal of tissue or a fluid sample for microscopic examination.

Pathologist

A physician who makes the diagnosis of lymphoma and other cancers from evaluating biopsies and other surgical specimens under the microscope.

Gastrointestinal tract

The gut, from mouth to anus.

9. What is the difference between Hodgkin lymphoma and non-Hodgkin lymphoma?

The two main types of lymphoma are **Hodgkin lymphoma** and **non-Hodgkin lymphoma**. Hodgkin lymphoma is named after Thomas Hodgkin, an English pathologist who originally described the disease in 1832.

Hodgkin lymphoma is a cancer of the lymphatic system that arises from a B-lymphocyte. There are two broad categories of Hodgkin lymphoma. The first is classical Hodgkin lymphoma, which includes 4 different subtypes (see **Table 1**). The second, less-common type is lymphocyte-predominant Hodgkin lymphoma, which tends to occur in older individuals. The distinction between these categories and between Hodgkin and non-Hodgkin lymphoma is made by careful pathological evaluation of lymph nodes. Hodgkin lymphoma most commonly affects people in their late teens or early 20s and in their 50s.

Non-Hodgkin lymphomas also arise most commonly from B-lymphocytes, but these lymphomas also from T lymphocytes and NK cells. Non-Hodgkin lymphomas generally increase in incidence with age. There are many different types of non-Hodgkin lymphoma, which are discussed later.

Hodgkin lymphoma

A type of lymphoma.

Non-Hodgkin lymphoma

The most common type of lymphoma.

Table 1 The different types of Hodgkin lymphoma

Type	Prevalence
Nodular sclerosing	Most common (75%)
Lymphocyte predominant	
Mixed cellularity	
Lymphocyte depleted	Least common (less than 5%)

10. What are the symptoms of lymphoma?

The most common presentation of a lymphoma is the finding of enlarged or swollen lymph nodes (**lymphadenopathy**) by the patient or a physician. They are commonly found initially in the neck, armpit, or groin, as these are areas where superficial lymph nodes can easily be felt when enlarged (**Table 2**). The enlarged lymph nodes are usually painless, but may be tender if they have grown very quickly. The most common cause of an enlarged lymph node is an infection, which is much more likely to cause the node to be tender. Most frequently, enlarged lymph nodes within the chest or abdomen do not cause any symptoms at all.

Lymphadenopathy

Enlarged lymph nodes.

The lymphatic system branches throughout the body, so these areas of lymphatic swelling may occur virtually anywhere. Lymph node enlargement can result in pressure effects on nearby structures. For example lymph node enlargement in the groin or the axilla can occasionally result in swelling of the leg or arm on the same side. If the lymph node swelling develops in or around your stomach area or intestinal tract, you may have abdominal pain and/or bloating, or a feeling of getting full faster than normal when eating. When the lymph nodes in the chest become involved, cough, shortness of breath, or chest pain may develop. If the lymph nodes in the center of the chest get big very quickly, they can sometimes cause **superior vena cava syndrome**, which is a slowing of blood flow returning to your heart from your arms and head, resulting from pressure on veins by the lymph nodes. This can result in headache, swelling (possibly affecting the head, neck, and arms), difficulty breathing, or vision problems.

Superior vena cava syndrome

A condition in which the blood flow back to the heart is decreased due to obstruction, usually by very large lymph nodes.

Table 2 Symptoms Associated with Lymphoma

Lymphoma symptoms are not specific. Not all people with lymphoma will experience all symptoms, and some will have symptoms not listed here. Common symptoms may include:

- Fatigue
- Painless swelling of lymph glands
- Fevers
- Night sweats
- Weight loss

If bone marrow is involved, you may experience anemia that results in generalized weakness and **fatigue**. Bleeding may result from a low platelet count, or infections may occur as a result of a low white blood cell count. Occasionally, lymphoma can also involve the brain or spinal cord, resulting in headaches, double vision, or weakness in an arm or leg. With involvement of the spinal cord, back pain, leg weakness, numbness, or problems related to the control of bowel or bladder function may occur. Most commonly, the spinal cord itself is not involved, but the lymphoma may press on the spinal cord, resulting in these problems. If any symptoms of spinal cord involvement occur, you should see your doctor immediately or, at night, go to the emergency room, as any delay could result in paralysis.

Other symptoms that can occur, regardless of the site of the lymphoma, may include fever, night sweats, and weight loss (these are the **B symptoms**); when these symptoms are present to a significant degree, they indicate a more aggressive lymphoma.

Many people with lymphoma won't have any symptoms. In these cases, the enlarged lymph nodes may be felt in the shower or while lying in bed. Occasionally, your

Fatigue

Tiredness, particularly the debilitating, continuous tiredness that signals illness or disease.

B symptoms

Fevers, night sweats, and weight loss that may occur in lymphoma patients. They can occur individually or together.

Indolent

Slow growing.

physician may detect them during a routine physical examination; this is more common with the **indolent** lymphomas.

Another important point to remember is that no symptoms are unique to lymphoma. Most of the time, symptoms from something other than lymphoma will be seen. In most people with enlarged, painful lymph nodes, various infections are a much more common cause, but if the lymph node remains large or continues to grow, especially if it is not painful, you should see your physician, who should consider a biopsy.

Before the biopsy, usually performed by a surgeon, your primary care doctor will have carried out a careful medical history, a physical examination, some blood tests, and perhaps some X-rays or scans.

11. How is lymphoma diagnosed?

The diagnosis of lymphoma is usually made from a lymph node biopsy. This involves obtaining an abnormal lymph node or a piece of an abnormal lymph node and examining it under a microscope. It is important to understand in the vast majority of cases the purpose of the biopsy is only to make a diagnosis. Except in very unique situations (e.g., a very localized indolent lymphoma) a biopsy is not meant to be a "treatment" per se for a lymphoma. Before the biopsy, usually performed by a surgeon, your primary care doctor will have carried out a careful medical history, a physical examination, some blood tests, and perhaps some X-rays or scans.

Lymph node architecture

The structure of lymph nodes when they are seen under a microscope.

It is generally preferable that an entire lymph node be removed (an excisional biopsy) when a lymphoma is suspected. This is because the appearance and distribution of the abnormal cells in the node (referred to as the **lymph node architecture**) are sometimes clues to the diagnosis of a lymphoma or may help in determining the subtype of lymphoma. If the lymph node is very large, it is possible that only a portion of it may need to be removed (an incisional biopsy) to obtain sufficient tissue to make a diagnosis. In situations where the only abnormal lymph node(s) is/are deep in the body, a radiologist may be asked to perform a special type of needle biopsy known as a core needle biopsy using ultrasound or computerized tomography (CT or CAT) scan images to guide the biopsy. This biopsy produces a small core of tissue with minimal risks and a reasonable chance of making a diagnosis successfully. This spares the patient a larger operation. However the core needle biopsy produces a smaller piece of tissue than that obtained with an excisional or incisional biopsy and occasionally this may not be enough tissue to establish the diagnosis or more likely the exact subtype of lymphoma if it is a lymphoma. The risk versus benefit of each type of biopsy must be considered when making the decision. Very rarely a physician may wish to start with a very small biopsy known as **fine needle aspiration (FNA)**. This is easier to do and less invasive than a core biopsy or excisional/incisional biopsy. However, for the purposes of diagnosing the lymphoma, it is rarely sufficient, although it may establish that the cells are lymphocytes rather than some other type of cell that may suggest a different disorder. In our opinion a patient in whom a lymphoma is strongly suspected should forego a fine needle aspiration and proceed to one of the other procedures described above. Your doctors will decide which type is best, depending on the size and location of the node. The decision is made in part on the basis of the structures that are around the nodes (e.g., blood vessels or nerves), since a biopsy could be associated with some risk of damaging those surrounding tissues. The biopsy is usually performed in the doctor's office or in the hospital and, depending on which part of the body is involved, can be done with either a local or general anesthetic.

Fine needle aspiration (FNA)

A procedure to obtain a sample of tissue using a small needle.

After removal, the lymph node is sent to the laboratory, where the lymph node tissue is treated with special chemicals to "fix" it, which results in preservation of the tissue. Then it is cut into very thin sections, placed on glass slides, and stained, making it ready for the pathologist to examine. The staining allows the different cells and structures within the lymph node to be distinguished from one another.

The pathologist examines the lymph node to see whether the cells are normal or abnormal. It is common for lymph nodes to become enlarged in reaction to infection or inflammation, in which case the findings are **benign**. If it is **malignant**, it can be either lymphoma or a different type of cancer that began somewhere else and has spread to a nearby lymph node.

Benign

Not cancerous.

Malignant

Cancerous.

After the pathologist has decided that it is lymphoma, distinguishing between Hodgkin lymphoma and non-Hodgkin lymphoma becomes important. The types of cells and their pattern under the microscope are most helpful for this purpose. Immunohistochemistry (antibody staining of the tissue on the pathology slides) is often used to distinguish the different types of lymphoma, as cells from many different types of lymphoma can appear similar under the microscope.

Flow cytometry

A procedure for examining the proteins present on the surface of cells.

Another helpful test called **flow cytometry** provides an additional way of examining and identifying different types of cells by looking at the pattern of particular proteins that exist on their surface. Different lymphomas have particular patterns of protein expression that help to determine the exact type of lymphoma. Flow cytometry or immunohistochemistry will be performed in almost all cases in which lymphoma is suspected. It is helpful to think of these tests as providing a fingerprint of the protein pattern on the surface of the cells, telling the pathologist that a group of identical abnormal cells are present, and assisting the pathologist in making an exact determination of what kind of lymphoma is present in the tissue.

As you will see, given that there are so many different types of lymphoma and the differences between many of them can be very subtle, it can sometimes be very difficult to be sure of the type of lymphoma that one has. In these rare cases, it is a good idea to get a second opinion from another pathologist. This is especially true if knowing the exact type will change the way the lymphoma will be treated. In many cases, the difference is so subtle that it will not affect the treatment, and from a practical point of view, the distinction is less important.

12. Could my lymphoma have been diagnosed earlier, and would it have made a difference?

When a lump is first discovered, depending on the circumstances and its characteristics, the internist or family doctor may want to keep an eye on the lump, as most lumps are due to benign (i.e., not cancerous) causes and go away without specific treatment. In the vast majority of cases, the swelling may be due to infection or inflammation, and the doctor might prescribe antibiotics. If the lump is suspected to be from a viral illness, observation may be sufficient initially since antibiotics don't treat viral illnesses; rather your normal immune system will resolve it over days to a few weeks. Often, a biopsy will be considered only if the lump persists or grows over a few weeks or has initial features suggesting the possibility of cancer.

However, if you find out that you have a lymphoma instead of an infection, it is natural to wonder why the diagnosis was not made sooner and whether the delay in diagnosis will have an effect on your outcome. Most doctors will not hesitate to discuss your concerns about the timing of the diagnosis; if this is not done, your questions may linger and distract you from coping with everything else that is happening. If all patients with a lump subsequently found not to be lymphoma were subjected to a biopsy, many unnecessary biopsies would be performed.

The question of whether diagnosing the lymphoma earlier makes a difference can be complicated. Lymphoma is very different from other cancers (such as breast, bowel, or lung cancer) in this respect. In these and other cancers, the ability to cure the disease largely depends on whether the cancer has spread from the site where it initially started. This is not generally true for lymphoma for a couple of reasons. First, the lymphatic system where the cancer begins is distributed throughout the body, meaning lymphoma cells generally have easy access to several sites in the body through the bloodstream and lymphatic vessels. These are normal everyday routes of travel for many types of lymphocytes. The lymphoma cells therefore may have spread fairly far from the place the lymphoma originated from very early on, when the disease was still microscopic and undetectable because that was a normal characteristic of that type of cell. Second, lymphoma cells are generally much more sensitive to chemotherapy drugs than most other types of cancer, meaning they can still generally be treated effectively and, in some cases, even cured at more advanced stages. Therefore spreading from one place to another does not necessarily have the same ominous implications as it does in other types of cancer. The ability to cure lymphoma depends more on what particular type of lymphoma you have—whether it is indolent or aggressive rather than whether it is in only one spot. That is not to say that having a lymphoma confined to one or two areas is not a better situation than having a lymphoma that is more widespread; nevertheless, lymphoma that has spread can also be treated effectively.

13. What causes lymphoma?

The cause of lymphoma in most people remains unknown. No definite association has been made with smoking or alcohol. Particular diets or lifestyles in general do not appear to increase the chance of developing lymphoma. Lymphoma does not occur as a result of previous injury to parts of the body. There is also an increased incidence of lymphoma associated with massive obesity. Smoking, alcohol and obesity have been associated with worse survival following a diagnosis of lymphoma for reasons that are not presently understood. Lymphoma can't spread from one person to another. Based on the increased incidence in association with immunodeficiency or inflammation including autoimmune disorders, it is felt that chronic immunologic stimulation of lymphocytes plays a role in the development of many types of lymphoma.

Many scientists have tried to identify certain things that could cause lymphoma. In most cases, the evidence for an association is weak, although exposure to certain chemicals such as insecticides or pesticides over prolonged periods of time may result in a higher incidence of lymphoma. These chemicals have been implicated in a higher incidence of non-Hodgkin lymphoma among farm workers in some rural areas of the US.

It is very clear that an abnormal immune system increases the chances of developing lymphoma.

Acquired immunodeficiency syndrome (AIDS)

The syndrome resulting from infection with the human immunodeficiency virus (HIV).

Human immunodeficiency virus (HIV)

A virus that attacks the human immune system, leaving the carrier prone to infections.

Sjögren's syndrome

An autoimmune disorder causing inflammation of the salivary and lacrimal (tear) glands, resulting in dry eyes and a dry mouth.

It is very clear that an abnormal immune system increases the chances of developing lymphoma. The most dramatic example of this is **acquired immunodeficiency syndrome (AIDS)**, caused by the **human immunodeficiency virus (HIV)**. This virus infects lymphocytes, resulting in depletion of CD4 helper cells, which are a particular type of T-lymphocyte. This results in a markedly abnormal immune system. Historically, this patient population developed lymphomas at a rate much higher than expected for the population in general. With the subsequent development and introduction of highly active antiretroviral therapy (HAART), the incidence of lymphoma in patients with HIV infection has fallen dramatically suggesting the importance of a well-functioning immune system in at least some aspects of the development of lymphoma. Individuals who undergo heart, lung, kidney, or liver transplants have a higher incidence of lymphoma. These organ transplant recipients have a lifelong requirement to take medicine to prevent rejection of the transplanted organ. The antirejection drugs impair many aspects of the organ recipient's normal immune function and this is very likely the reason for the increased risk of lymphomas in patients who have received organ transplants. These types of lymphomas are often referred to collectively as posttransplant lymphoproliferative disorders (PTLD). It is generally non-Hodgkin lymphoma that occurs, but sometimes Hodgkin lymphoma is also seen. Some types of PTLDs may shrink or regress with a decrease in the dose of antirejection medicine, suggesting that allowing the patient's immune system to regain some additional function may assist in the control of the PTLD.

Autoimmune diseases are associated with an increased risk of the development of lymphoma. The most common reported associations have been with **Sjögren's syndrome** (parotid lymphomas), autoimmune thyroiditis (thyroid lymphomas), rheumatoid arthritis and **Systemic lupus erythematosus**. The incidence of T-cell lymphoma has been reported to be higher in patients with celiac disease and psoriasis. The chronic stimulation of the immune system that occurs with these disorders or the immunosuppressive medicines that are used to treat the autoimmune disease likely both contribute to the apparent increased risk of lymphoma in these settings. Since patients with more severe disease require more powerful treatment, it is very difficult to separate out the effect of the disorder versus the effect of the treatment, but both appear to play a role in the development of lymphomas under these circumstances.

Another virus that has been implicated as a cause of lymphoma is the **Epstein-Barr virus (EBV)**, which infects many people without causing any illness and is also the cause of infectious mononucleosis (popularly known as "glandular fever" or "mono," and often called "the kissing disease," as it is common among adolescents and is spread through **saliva**). Once the virus gains entrance into the body it remains there virtually forever, eventually becoming inactive (dormant) in B lymphocytes. It has been shown that the virus can insert itself into the genes in B cells that normally control growth and division of cells. It is conceivable that if the virus came out of its dormant state, such as might occur in people with immune deficiency, it could affect those genes and send signals telling the cell to start to divide. In the laboratory, this virus can make B-lymphocytes grow abnormally. Some lymphoma patients have EBV present in their lymphoma cells, suggesting that the virus may be involved in the development of their lymphoma; however, another explanation is that the immune abnormality that allowed the lymphoma to develop also allowed

Systemic lupus erythematosus

A disease in which the immune system attacks the body, causing inflammatory damage to multiple organs, including the skin, kidneys, heart, or brain.

Epstein-Barr virus (EBV)

The virus that causes infectious mononucleosis and can cause lymphocytes to grow abnormally.

Saliva

The lubricating substance produced by the salivary glands that is essential for chewing and swallowing.

DIAGNOSIS AND CLASSIFICATION OF LYMPHOMA

the EBV infection to occur. This would make EBV an innocent bystander infection rather than the cause of the lymphoma. Currently, the treatment of lymphoma is usually not different whether EBV is or is not present. Therefore, testing is not done on a routine basis. An exception to this is when lymphoma occurs after organ transplantation, when testing for EBV may be important and treatment potentially influenced by the presence of EBV.

An unusual type of lymphoma occurs in some people infected with the **human T-cell lymphotropic virus type 1 (HTLV-1)**. This virus occurs most frequently in Japan and parts of the Caribbean, and can result in a form of T-cell lymphoma that can be very aggressive but fortunately is quite rare.

Human T-cell lymphotropic virus type 1 (HTLV-1)

A virus that can cause leukemia by infecting T lymphocytes.

The **hepatitis C virus** appears to increase the chances of developing lymphoma. This is worrisome, as the number of people infected with this virus has increased dramatically over the past 20 years. Hepatitis C infection has been associated with the development of cryoglobulinemia, sometimes a precursor to lymphoma. It has also been associated with the development of aggressive lymphomas, including **diffuse large B-cell lymphoma (DLBCL)**. There are also reports that hepatitis C, like *Helicobacter pylori*, has been associated with extranodal **marginal zone lymphoma** of the stomach as well as lymphoma of the spleen and liver as well as follicular lymphoma.

Hepatitis C virus

One of the viruses that can infect the liver and cause chronic liver inflammation.

Diffuse large B-cell lymphoma (DLBCL)

A type of intermediate-grade lymphoma.

Marginal zone lymphoma

A type of indolent lymphoma.

Yet another virus associated with lymphoma is the human herpesvirus 8 (HHV8). Another name for this virus is Kaposi's sarcoma herpesvirus. It has been associated with a particular type of lymphoma called primary effusion lymphoma (PEL). This is a lymphoma originally diagnosed in AIDS patients, but it is occasionally seen in non–HIV-infected patients. It usually presents with fluid around the lung or heart, or in the abdominal cavity.

Helicobacter pylori is an interesting bacterium that causes lymphoma in some patients. This bacterium has also been associated with the development of stomach cancer. Most often, this bacterium causes chronic inflammation in the form of gastritis and does not go on to cause any type of cancer. The type of lymphoma associated with *Helicobacter pylori* is usually an extranodal marginal zone lymphoma of the stomach, and, when it is still localized to the stomach, it may respond to antibiotic therapy.

In the prior examples of associations between infectious agents and lymphomas, the observation that treating the infection sometimes causes regression of the lymphoma is evidence that the infection is still "driving" the existence of that particular lymphoma. It suggests that those lymphomas are still dependent on the presence of the infection for their existence, and that they have not quite yet begun to grow independent of the infection. These lymphomas can sometimes subsequently acquire new genetic abnormalities (mutations) within them that cause them to "break away" from the infection as a driving force and grow independent of the infection at which point treating the infection will not shrink the lymphoma. At this point conventional types of treatment are required.

14. How is lymphoma classified?

It is important to understand that although lymphomas are threats to the health of the person affected, they are also disorders that, in a sense, occur as a natural consequence of our imperfect human biology. As such, any classification system that tries to place such a wide variety of biologic occurrences into perfect little "boxes" that we can name (diagnose) will be an imperfect system with occasional gaps and occasional overlap in certain entities. There are now over 70 different types of lymphoma described. Historically, in order to make sense of the different types, a classification system was necessary. The fundamental classification is between Hodgkin lymphoma and non-Hodgkin lymphoma (see **Table 3**). For non-Hodgkin lymphomas, there have been a number of different classifications used over the years. These include the Rappaport, Kiel, Lukes-Collins, **Working Formulation, Revised European-American Lymphoma Classification (REAL)**, and most recently, the World Health Organization (WHO) Classification. The Working Formulation introduced in the early 1980s classified lymphomas into low grade, intermediate grade, and high grade based on the appearance of the lymphoma cells under the microscope and their clinical behavior. As a greater understanding of lymphoma has developed and newer technology (e.g., flow cytometry, immunohistochemistry, molecular tests) to evaluate proteins on the surface of lymphoma cells and genetic changes occurring within the cells has become available, a much greater ability to distinguish between similar types of lymphoma has emerged. This has resulted in the need for more sophisticated and helpful classification systems and ultimately led to the development of the WHO classification. The updated 2008 classification was introduced to replace the original 2001 WHO Lymphoma Classification. This resulted from new information emerging over recent years. There was also emerging information about specific types of lymphoma occurring in younger and older people as well as more particular lymphomas related to the presence of immune suppression. This allowed better separation

Working formulation

One of the lymphoma classifications.

Revised European-American Classification (REAL)

The basis of the newest lymphoma classification.

and classification of lymphomas that had previously been listed together. In earlier classifications, aggressive B-cell lymphomas had been listed as DLBCL. In the latest version, there are a number of new types of lymphoma listed under the aggressive category, as opposed to them all being lumped together as DLBCL.

Appropriate classification is also very important for conducting clinical trials, where it is important to identify groups of patients with a similar type of lymphoma. This allows for the development and evaluation of treatments specifically geared toward the type of lymphoma studied.

In the current WHO classification, individual types of non-Hodgkin lymphoma are listed according to a number of features, including the cell of origin (B cell, T cell, or NK cell), appearance under the microscope, types of protein present on the surface of the cells, genetic features, and clinical features. It is useful in clinical practice to consider groups of these entities according to whether they behave in an indolent fashion or an aggressive fashion. This is the way lymphoma was classified in previous classifications. As this is still an important point in considering lymphoma, the table from the previous classification is shown in **Table 4**. All this information is then used to determine the appropriate type of therapy or, if one is considering a clinical trial, ensuring that appropriate patients are enrolled into that clinical trial.

For Hodgkin lymphoma, there are two broad categories. These include classical Hodgkin lymphoma and nodular lymphocyte–predominant Hodgkin lymphoma (NLPHL). Classical Hodgkin lymphoma is further classified into four types, also shown in Table 3.

DIAGNOSIS AND CLASSIFICATION OF LYMPHOMA

Table 3 Classification of non-Hodgkin lymphoma and Hodgkin lymphoma

The mature B-cell neoplasms

Chronic lymphocytic leukemia/small lymphocytic lymphoma

B-cell prolymphocytic leukemia

Splenic marginal zone lymphoma

Hairy cell leukemia

Splenic lymphoma/leukemia, unclassifiable

    Splenic diffuse red pulp small B-cell lymphoma*

    Hairy cell leukemia-variant*

Lymphoplasmacytic lymphoma

    Waldenström macroglobulinemia

Heavy chain diseases

    Alpha heavy chain disease

    Gamma heavy chain disease

    Mu heavy chain disease

Plasma cell myeloma

Solitary plasmacytoma of bone

Extraosseous plasmacytoma

Extranodal marginal zone B-cell lymphoma of mucosa-associated lymphoid tissue (MALT lymphoma)

Nodal marginal zone B-cell lymphoma (MZL)

    Pediatric type nodal MZL

Follicular lymphoma

    Pediatric type follicular lymphoma

Primary cutaneous follicle center lymphoma

Mantle cell lymphoma

Diffuse large B-cell lymphoma (DLBCL), not otherwise specified

    T cell/histiocyte rich large B-cell lymphoma

    DLBCL associated with chronic inflammation

    Epstein-Barr virus (EBV) + DLBCL of the elderly

Lymphomatoid granulomatosis

Primary mediastinal (thymic) large B-cell lymphoma

Intravascular large B-cell lymphoma

* designates provisional entities

Primary cutaneous DLBCL, leg type

ALK+ large B-cell lymphoma

Plasmablastic lymphoma

Primary effusion lymphoma

Large B-cell lymphoma arising in HHV8-associated multicentric Castleman disease

Burkitt lymphoma

B-cell lymphoma, unclassifiable, with features intermediate between diffuse large B-cell lymphoma and Burkitt lymphoma

B-cell lymphoma, unclassifiable, with features intermediate between diffuse large B-cell lymphoma and classical Hodgkin lymphoma

The mature T-cell and NK-cell neoplasms

T-cell prolymphocytic leukemia

T-cell large granular lymphocytic leukemia

Chronic lymphoproliferative disorder of NK-cells

Aggressive NK cell leukemia

Systemic EBV+ T-cell lymphoproliferative disease of childhood (associated with chronic active EBV infection)

Hydroa vacciniforme-like lymphoma

Adult T-cell leukemia/ lymphoma Extranodal

NK/T-cell lymphoma, nasal type

Enteropathy-associated T-cell lymphoma

Hepatosplenic T-cell lymphoma

Subcutaneous panniculitis-like T-cell lymphoma

Mycosis fungoides

Sézary syndrome

Primary cutaneous CD30+ T-cell lymphoproliferative disorder

    Lymphomatoid papulosis

      Primary cutaneous anaplastic large-cell lymphoma

Primary cutaneous aggressive epidermotropic CD8+ cytotoxic T-cell lymphoma*

Primary cutaneous gamma-delta T-cell lymphoma

Primary cutaneous small/medium CD4+ T-cell lymphoma*

(continues)

* designates provisional entities

Table 3 Classification of non-Hodgkin lymphoma and
Hodgkin lymphoma (continued)

Peripheral T-cell lymphoma, not otherwise specified

Angioimmunoblastic T-cell lymphoma

Anaplastic large cell lymphoma (ALCL), ALK+

Anaplastic large cell lymphoma (ALCL), ALK–

Hodgkin lymphoma

Nodular lymphocyte predominant Hodgkin lymphoma.

Classical Hodgkin lymphoma

    Nodular sclerosis

    Mixed cellularity

    Lymphocyte depleted

    Lymphocyte rich

* designates provisional entities

Table 4 Previous WHO classification of non-Hodgkin lymphoma

Indolent	Aggressive
B cell	**B cell**
Small lymphocytic lymphoma/ Chronic Lymphocytic Leukemia	Follicular lymphoma grade 3
Lymphoplasmacytic lymphoma	Diffuse large B-cell lymphoma
Follicular lymphoma grade 1 and 2	Mantle cell lymphoma*
Marginal zone B-cell lymphoma	Burkitt lymphoma**
Mantle cell lymphoma*	Lymphoblasic lymphoma**
T cell	**T cell**
Mycosis fungoides	Peripheral T-cell lymphoma
	Anaplastic large cell lymphoma
	Adult T-cell leukemia/lymphoma**
	Lymphoblastic lymphoma**

*Mantle cell lymphoma can behave as an indolent or an aggressive lymphoma.

**These lymphomas are highly aggressive.

15. How is lymphoma staged?

Both Hodgkin lymphoma and non-Hodgkin lymphoma are staged in similar ways. There are four possible **stages** (see **Table 5**) based on the extent of the lymphoma throughout the body and whether there is involvement of organs outside the lymph node system. Each stage can be further divided into A or B, depending on the presence (B) or absence (A) of unexplained fevers, drenching night sweats, and weight loss (see Question 10 on page 20 for more on symptoms). In general, the presence of B symptoms is more commonly associated with higher-grade lymphomas and/or higher stages of lymphoma.

A group of lymphoma experts (meeting in Ann Arbor, Michigan, in 1971) devised the staging system for Hodgkin lymphoma known as the **Ann Arbor Staging System**. Since then, it has been applied very successfully to non-Hodgkin lymphoma and remains the best staging system available for both Hodgkin lymphoma and non-Hodgkin lymphoma.

Stage

A reference to the number of places in the body affected by lymphoma or other cancer.

Ann Arbor Staging System

Used to describe the areas in the body affected by the lymphoma. It was created at a conference held in Ann Arbor, Michigan.

Table 5 Staging of Lymphoma*

Stage I	One lymph node area involved
Stage II	Involvement of two or more lymph node areas on the same side of the diaphragm
Stage III	Lymph nodes involved on both sides of the diaphragm
Stage IV	Any of the above with involvement of sites other than lymph nodes (most commonly the bone marrow, liver, or lungs)
B symptoms	Fever, night sweats, or significant weight loss

*After designation of the stage based on the sites of involvement, patients are categorized as either A (if no B symptoms are present) or B (if B symptoms are present).

Staging is very important information for every patient with lymphoma, as it provides a common language for doctors and patients to describe the areas affected within the body and its overall extent. With few exceptions (e.g., cutaneous T-cell lymphomas), the same staging system is used for virtually all lymphomas. It is vital information for deciding on the correct treatment and can also be helpful in estimating your **prognosis**.

Prognosis

A prediction of the course that a disease will take.

As noted, there are four stages described in the Ann Arbor system (the staging system uses Roman numerals). In this way, lymphoma can be designated as limited for stages I and II and more extensive for stages III and IV.

Stage I refers to involvement of a single lymph node region. Stage II refers to two or more lymph node regions, with the affected regions occurring on the same side of the **diaphragm** (the large muscle that separates the chest from the abdomen and is important for breathing). Stage III is designated by involvement of the lymph node regions on both sides of the diaphragm. (For the purposes of staging, the spleen is included as a lymph node region.) Stage IV includes involvement of disease not only in lymph node regions, but also in non–lymph node sites such as the bone marrow, liver, lungs, gut, or skin.

Diaphragm

The large muscle that separates the lungs from the abdomen. Its movement is important for breathing.

The presence of lymphoma involving a site other than the lymph nodes or spleen generally implies stage IV unless the involvement is felt to represent direct spread from a nearby lymph node. For example, if there is involvement of the lung directly next to involved lymph nodes in the chest, the subscript E is written beside the stage. In the previously mentioned example, stage II_E would indicate that the lymphoma involves more than one region on the same side of the diaphragm (i.e., stage II) and that the second area is felt to represent lymphoma which has extended directly or contiguously (i.e., an "E" designation) from a the adjacent lymph node into the lung tissue. Stage IV refers to lymphoma diffusely involving a non-lymphoid organ such as the bone marrow, liver, or lung, where it is not directly spreading from a lymph node. Although not stated explicitly in the staging descriptions, stage IV lymphoma generally implies that the lymphoma cells spread to the affected organ through the blood stream (i.e., hematogenously) rather than as a direct growth extension from a nearby lymph node.

Until about 20 years ago, many people with lymphoma underwent a surgical procedure called a **laparotomy** for staging. This procedure involved opening the abdomen, taking samples or biopsies of many lymph nodes, performing a liver biopsy, and removing the spleen. The spleen, lymph node, and liver biopsies would then be examined under a microscope to determine whether there was involvement by lymphoma. This surgical staging procedure was performed mostly in patients with limited-stage Hodgkin lymphoma but also in some patients with non-Hodgkin lymphoma. Prior to the widespread availability of high quality imaging tests such as **computed tomography (CT)** and more recently **positron emission tomography (PET) scans**, pathologic examination of multiple lymph node groups was felt to be the most accurate way to determine stage and generate a proper treatment plan. Today, with the wide availability of high-quality CT and PET scans for staging lymphomas, staging laparotomies have become a part of history

Staging now relies on the cumulative data gathered by performing a history and physical examination plus

Laparotomy

Surgery involving an incision to look directly into the abdomen.

Computed tomography (CT) scan

A specialized type of X-ray that creates a detailed cross-sectional view of the body.

Positron emission tomography (PET) scan

X-ray studies that use the abnormal sugar metabolism of cancer cells to identify metastatic deposits.

high-quality imaging studies such as CT scans, PET scans, or both, along with a bone marrow biopsy/ examination (**Table 6**).

The physical examination for staging focuses on determining whether there is enlargement of the lymph nodes, liver, and spleen. On examination, enlarged lymph nodes in the head and neck region, the armpit (axilla), and also the groin (inguinal region) can be detected. Lymph nodes are occasionally felt in the elbow or knee region. In order for the spleen to be felt, it needs to be two to three times larger than normal. The radiologic studies mentioned above are especially helpful for detecting lymph node enlargement internally that cannot be felt on examination. These include the lymph nodes between the lungs (hilar and **mediastinal nodes**) and the lymph nodes in the abdomen (**retroperitoneal** and **mesenteric lymph nodes**). In people without lymphoma, lymph nodes are normally present at these sites but are not enlarged, usually measuring up to only 1 cm in size.

A bone marrow examination is a very important part of the staging evaluation. Historically this test was sometimes done on both sides of the hipbone (a bilateral biopsy), but with improvements in other staging tests as well as technical improvements in finding lymphoma cells in the marrow this test is not performed commonly on both sides of the hipbone today.

Mediastinal nodes

Lymph nodes present in the area between the lungs.

Retroperitoneal lymph nodes

The most common lymph nodes present in the abdomen.

Mesenteric lymph nodes

The lymph nodes present in the abdomen tissue that anchors the bowel.

Magnetic resonance imaging (MRI)

A technique based on the use of magnetic fields to produce images of body parts.

Table 6 Tests for staging of lymphoma

Tests necessary for staging	Tests sometimes required
Physical examination	Bone marrow biopsy on both sides
PET/CT scan	Spinal tap
Bone marrow biopsy	MRI* scan

*MRI = magnetic resonance imagings

The most commonly used radiologic tests for staging are the CT scan and the PET scan (see Question 16 on page 43). A CT scan may be done on its own in which case the patient is generally given **contrast dye** both to drink and as an injection into the vein. A specialized dough-nut shaped X-ray camera spins around the patient taking many individual pictures at different angles, and these are then combined into multiple, computer-generated, cross-sectional images at each level of the body that needs to be examined. Such scans are commonly performed on the neck, chest, abdomen, and pelvis. The contrast dyes given for this type of CT scan create better visual dis-tinction between the lymph nodes and other tissues, including blood vessels and gut; however, the dye can occasionally affect kidney function. The contrast dye can also cause allergic reactions. Patients who develop aller-gies to the contrast dye can still generally receive contrast if they are premedicated with a small to moderate dose of steroids prior to receiving the dye injection. If your doctor feels that the risk of the contrast outweighs its benefits, a non-contrast CT scan or a combination PET/CT scan may be ordered. CT scans are very good for examin-ing the size and structure of lymph nodes and organs, but cannot always determine definitively whether or not lymph nodes or organs contain lymphoma especially when they are not enlarged or abnormal in their appear-ance on the scan. The advantage of a PET scan is that it can often suggest the presence of lymphoma in lymph nodes or other structures that are still normal in size and radiographic appearance (see Question 16). However not all types of lymphoma are well visualized by PET and as such PET scans are not always the best staging test for a lymphoma. At the time of diagnosis, if a lymph node biopsy confirms lymphoma, it is reasonable to assume that other enlarged lymph nodes are also involved with lymphoma; however, after treatment, lymph nodes can

Contrast dye

A chemical that is injected for certain X-rays, including CT scans and MRI scans, that results in better contrast pictures.

The most com-monly used radiologic tests for staging are the CT scan and the PET scan.

remain enlarged due to large amounts of inflammation or scar tissue and not due to residual lymphoma. These nodes may still look big on a CT scan but may not contain active residual lymphoma. This limitation of the CT is largely what drove the need for so-called "functional imaging" tests such as the **gallium scans** and PET scans. Gallium scans are rarely used in the US since PET scans are generally widely available and are perceived as providing more information about the lymphoma.

A **lymphangiogram** is an older test that is no longer performed today but is of some historical interest. It was a technically a difficult test for the radiologist to perform and few radiologists practicing today are likely to have any experience in either performing or interpreting the test. The procedure involves injecting dye into the lymph vessels of both feet. These vessels are very tiny and difficult to find. Once injected, the dye travels to the lymph nodes in the groin and abdomen and can show abnormal lymph nodes using X-rays even if they are not larger than normal. The test had been most useful for the accurate staging of Hodgkin lymphoma, but with the availability of high-quality CT scanning and the availability of PET or PET/CT scans, this test has become another part of history.

Accurate staging is a very important aspect of lymphoma management. It identifies patients who have early or so-called limited stage disease who may benefit from a different treatment approach than patients with more extensive disease. This is mostly true for patients with Hodgkin lymphoma, but to some extent is still applicable to non-Hodgkin lymphoma. This is because the main determinant of treatment and outcome in non-Hodgkin lymphoma is often the subtype of lymphoma, rather than the extent of involvement throughout the body.

Gallium scan

A nuclear medicine test that uses gallium to show areas of lymphoma within the body.

Lymphangiogram

An X-ray study of lymph glands after they are injected with a dye.

16. What is a positron emission tomography (PET) scan?

The PET scan involves injection of a small amount of radioactive glucose (sugar) into the bloodstream. Actively growing/dividing cells such as lymphoma cells pick up the glucose and can be imaged using a special camera. Therefore, even if the lymph nodes are not enlarged, a PET scan can potentially detect areas of suspected lymphoma. As stated previously, one of the most important advantages of a PET scan is that it can potentially detect lymphoma in lymph nodes that are minimally involved and still normal in size by exam or by CT scanning. A PET scan is very often combined with a CT scan to improve the accuracy of the scan. In these cases, the CT is usually done without contrast as described earlier. When a radiologist interprets a PET scan, they will be able to determine which sites in the body take up abnormal amounts of the radioactive glucose and how intense the glucose uptake is. The strength of this signal is often measured using something known as a standard uptake value (SUV). A very high SUV could raise the suspicion of transformation from a low-grade to a higher-grade lymphoma, but would generally need to be confirmed with a biopsy of the involved area. If proven, this would usually result in a change in therapy.

Unfortunately the PET/CT scan is not able to detect all bone marrow involvement and does not yet generally replace the need to do a bone marrow biopsy.

At the present time, the most established use of a PET scan is to determine if the lymphoma is in remission at the end of therapy, particularly for potentially curable lymphomas such as diffuse large-B cell lymphoma and Hodgkin lymphoma. Many other uses for PET are under consideration and are the subject of ongoing research. One example of another potential use of PET scans involves repeating a PET scan part of the way through therapy (often called an interim scan) to determine if the course of treatment could be changed (e.g., intensified, reduced in intensity, or shortened). Another example might be to decide if **radiation therapy** or even a repeat tissue biopsy is required at the end of chemotherapy treatments. All of these types of questions require more study to determine whether such use of a PET scan might change some aspects of therapy in the future. The vast majority of clinical trials selectively focusing on PET scan information today, particularly in Hodgkin lymphoma are directed at this question of altering the treatment strategy by obtaining an interim scan scan. It seems likely based on early results that these tests will alter our management of lymphomas in the coming years, but such studies will generally need to be mature (i.e., follow patients and results for a long time) and demonstrate repeatable (i.e., demonstrated in multiple trials) or very striking results to change the standard of care.

As stated previously, obtaining a PET following completion of treatment is very useful in determining whether or not certain types of lymphoma are in remission. A negative scan following treatment, for both Hodgkin lymphoma and non-Hodgkin lymphoma, indicates a very good chance of remaining in remission with a much lower risk of relapse. This is true even if the CT scan shows enlarged lymph nodes at the time of a negative PET scan.

Once a patient is in remission, questions are likely to arise regarding the value of periodic (often referred to

Radiation therapy

Treatment using radiation.

as surveillance) CT or PET scans to potentially detect a recurrence earlier than if it were brought to attention by a patient's symptoms, doctor's exam, or lab tests. This is a topic that can be difficult for patients to feel safe about and is best discussed with your personal physician. Although many physicians feel more comfortable recommending intermittent scans during follow-up, there is no clear evidence that finding a recurrence of lymphoma earlier improves the outcome after re-treatment. Additional considerations include the costs of testing, the repeated doses of radiation and dyes administered to the patient, and the possibility of the imaging studies falsely suggesting a problem (i.e., a false positive test result) where none really exists, leading to the perceived need for other tests and potentially biopsies which can occasionally result in complications such as bleeding or infection.

Generally at the time of a first recurrence of a lymphoma (e.g., by detection of an abnormal node or a new symptom that leads to a CT scan which is abnormal), a re-biopsy is required to prove whether or not it is a recurrence of lymphoma. Sometimes with indolent lymphomas, since they tend to recur repeatedly, a physician may not insist on a re-biopsy on the second or third recurrence unless there is a suspicion that the lymphoma has transformed or that it may be something other than a lymphoma. Also under certain circumstances evidence of progression/recurrence on a PET or CT (e.g., at a site previously known to be affected by lymphoma occurring a very short time after completion of prior therapy) may not require biopsy in the judgment of the physician. There is often no single right answer in most cases, and the decision to biopsy must be a shared decision with the patient and physician.

Thrombocytopenia

A low platelet count.

Leukopenia

A low white blood cell count.

Lymphoplasma-cytic lymphoma (LPL)

The lymphoma associated with Waldenstrom's macroglobulinemia.

Mantle cell lymphoma

An uncommon type of aggressive lymphoma.

Lymphoblastic lymphoma

An aggressive, fast-growing type of lymphoma.

Bone marrow sampling is important, as it affects the choice of treatment and is also frequently necessary for evaluating the response to treatment.

Dimples of Venus

The dimples seen on the skin over the sacrum on the lower back.

17. How is a bone marrow examination performed?

Evaluation of the bone marrow is a routine part of lymphoma staging. When bone marrow involvement occurs, production of all the normal blood cells may be decreased, resulting in a low red cell count (anemia), a low platelet count (**thrombocytopenia**), or a low white cell count (**leukopenia**). If there is lymphoma involvement in the bone marrow, the lymphoma is stage IV. Involvement of the bone marrow can occur with any type of lymphoma but is common in follicular lymphoma, grades 1 or 2, **lymphoplasmacytic lymphoma (LPL)**, **mantle cell lymphoma**, and **lymphoblastic lymphoma**. It is less common in Hodgkin lymphoma but, when present, can have a significant impact on the choice of treatment. Bone marrow involvement is not uncommon in DLBCL.

When staging lymphoma for the first time, a bone marrow sample occasionally may be obtained from both sides of the hip because only one side may contain the lymphoma. Bone marrow sampling is important, as it affects the choice of treatment and is also frequently necessary for evaluating the response to treatment.

The bone marrow is obtained from the hipbone at the back, generally at the site of the **dimples of Venus**, next to the tailbone. This procedure, usually done in 20 to 30 minutes in the outpatient clinic, can be done with the patient lying either on his or her side or front. The bone marrow test has two parts. The first is the bone marrow aspiration, which refers to the sampling of the liquid part of the bone marrow within the marrow cavity. This sample is good for looking at the size, shape, and features of individual cells. The second part of the test is the bone marrow biopsy, which involves taking a tiny core of the bone. When this is examined under the microscope, it shows a bird's eye view of the marrow within the bone. This is good for looking at the marrow architecture as well as the presence of lymphoma involvement.

First, the skin over the site on the hipbone is cleansed with a disinfectant and then numbed with local anesthetic, usually lidocaine. Next, the area down to the surface of the bone is numbed. The surface of the bone can be particularly sensitive when the lidocaine is first injected, as the lidocaine causes a stinging sensation. Next, a very small incision is made. The bone marrow needle is then advanced into the marrow cavity with a gentle corkscrew type of motion, which usually causes a sensation of pressure. The inside of the bone marrow is liquid, and a small amount (2 to 5 cc) is then sucked out with the needle. This only takes a couple of seconds, but for many people, it is the most uncomfortable part of the procedure. The bone marrow itself cannot be anesthetized, and when it is sucked out, it can feel like a very strange pulling sensation in the hip and also down the leg. The person doing the procedure can help by talking to you, describing each step, and giving you a warning before the marrow is withdrawn. This discomfort should only last a couple of seconds.

The second part of the test involves doing the biopsy. The biopsy needle is placed in the same area on the hip bone, and a hollow needle is advanced into the bone. Again, this should feel only like a pressure sensation. The needle is then removed with the piece of bone inside. Pressure is held over the site to prevent bleeding, and a bandage is applied to the area. This is the end of the procedure.

Although many centers offer the ability to have a bone marrow biopsy performed under heavy sedation (known as conscious sedation), many physicians feel that the use of this level of sedation is an excessive risk for the discomfort level associated with the biopsy itself. Also some institutions/physicians now use a kit that utilizes a battery powered device similar to a small drill that has been demonstrated to be a safe and effective alternative to the traditional needle device.

18. How do I prepare for a bone marrow test?

For many people, the worst part of the test is waiting for the appointment. The build-up of anxiety may actually increase the pain and discomfort associated with the test. Thus, a shorter appointment time may be helpful. If you are taking aspirin or a similar type of drug that prevents platelets from working properly, ask your doctor whether it should be stopped. Many patients find it helpful to have a friend or relative accompany them to the appointment. Usually a sedative is not necessary for the procedure, so patients can drive themselves to and from the appointment if necessary. In fact, many patients return to work after the test.

After the test, you can be up and about as normal. You may feel some aching discomfort in the area of the biopsy after the local anesthetic wears off, but this should only last for 1 or 2 days. A mild painkiller is usually effective in controlling the discomfort. Aspirin or similar medications are to be avoided, as they can increase the chance of bleeding. Bleeding from the site of the biopsy can occur, and simply applying pressure will generally stop most bleeding. It is very rare for an infection or serious bleeding to result from a bone marrow test.

19. What are the different types of non-Hodgkin lymphoma?

The classification of non-Hodgkin lymphoma is shown in Table 3 in Question 14 on page 31. The individual types of lymphoma have been classified either as indolent, aggressive or highly aggressive.

Indolent Non-Hodgkin Lymphoma

Indolent lymphomas generally are slow growing, and their characteristic appearance under the microscope generally provides the diagnosis. These lymphomas tend to respond well to therapy with patients often initially attaining long periods of remission, but eventually the lymphoma tends to recur. The indolent non-Hodgkin lymphomas are generally considered incurable with conventional types and doses of chemotherapy. At the time of diagnosis, the lymphoma is often stage IV, generally because the bone marrow as well as lymph nodes are involved. Circulating lymphoma cells may be seen in the bloodstream, and patients often have no symptoms.

Aggressive and Highly Aggressive Non-Hodgkin Lymphoma

These lymphomas include the group of lymphomas previously termed intermediate-grade and high-grade lymphomas. These lymphomas grow faster than the indolent lymphomas. They generally cause symptoms more rapidly and require the prompt institution of therapy. These lymphomas may present as stage I or II. This is in contrast to the indolent lymphomas, which frequently present as stage IV. Involvement of tissues or organs other than lymph nodes is also more common in this category of lymphoma.

DIAGNOSIS AND CLASSIFICATION OF LYMPHOMA

20. What are small lymphocytic lymphoma/chronic lymphocytic leukemia (SLL/CLL) and the related monoclonal B-cell lymphocytosis?

Monoclonal B-cell lymphocytosis (MBL) is the presence of low numbers of abnormal B-cells circulating in the blood. It is a relatively new concept/disorder as it has only recently been studied in people with normal or minimally abnormal blood counts. These cells may be found in approximately 5% of older individuals. The other blood counts should be normal and these individuals should not have any signs or symptoms of a hematologic disorder such as fevers, sweats, or enlarged lymph nodes or spleen. MBL is nothing that needs to be declared on any legal form. Generally it has been observed that individuals with MBL go on to develop some kind of lymphoma at a rate of 1–4% per year. The most common subsequent diagnosis that results from progression of MBCL is CLL/SLL or Waldenstrom's Macroglobulinema (see Question 21 on page 53). For most people, the only thing necessary is a repeat blood count. For those with very low numbers of abnormal B-cells, a repeat blood test should be performed at around 6 months to establish a stable count. Individuals with a higher abnormal B-cell count should have a blood count performed every year along with a physical examination, and should report any increased fatigue and any noticeable enlargement of lymph nodes or unexplained symptoms to their physician.

Small lymphocytic lymphoma (SLL) is very closely related to a type of chronic leukemia called **chronic lymphocytic leukemia (CLL)**. These disorders are so closely associated that they are grouped together in the current WHO **lymphoma classification**. Although

Small lymphocytic lymphoma (SLL)

A type of indolent lymphoma that is similar to chronic lymphocytic leukemia.

Chronic lymphocytic leukemia (CLL)

The most common slow-growing type of leukemia.

Lymphoma classification

A system to organize the many different types of lymphoma.

CLL is technically a type of "leukemia" the word leukemia simply refers to the presence of abnormal numbers of white blood cells in the circulation. Biologically CLL is a lymphoid disease that is for all intents and purposes just as easily considered a type of lymphoma. The "small" in the name refers to the size of the abnormal cells when seen under the microscope. This is generally a slow-growing lymphoma that occurs mostly in older people. At diagnosis, lymphoma involving the bone marrow is common, and most people are therefore in stage IV. The difference between the two diseases really depends on how many of the abnormal cells are present in the blood as compared with the lymph nodes. When relatively large numbers of cells are seen circulating in the bloodstream, it is called CLL. Although CLL is relatively common, this type of lymphoma is relatively rare, accounting for less than 5% of all non-Hodgkin lymphomas. The abnormal lymph nodes and blood/marrow both contain mature B-lymphocytes. It is unusual to have disease confined to the lymph nodes. Most patients will also have abnormal lymphocytes in the circulation. SLL is usually diagnosed after small, slow-growing lymph nodes are found. An abnormal blood test with a high white count consisting mostly of lymphocytes may also lead to the diagnosis. B symptoms are unusual. CLL/SLL are in some ways very similar to other indolent lymphomas, and in some ways very different. There is also often confusion about how to stage a patient who is said to have CLL (see below) versus a patient who is said to have SLL (where the usual Ann Arbor staging system would be used).

A very common staging system for CLL is known as the Rai staging system. This assigns a stage from 0- to 4 based on the following: 0: abnormal cells in the blood as the only sign of the illness; 1: the presence of enlarged lymph nodes (lymphadenopathy); 2: the presence of an enlarged liver and/or spleen; 3: low red cell count (anemia); 4: low platelets (thrombocytopenia). Stage 0 CLL is sometimes referred to as "low risk", stages 1–2 as "intermediate risk", and stages 3–4 as "high risk", although these terms can make patients feel misled, since stage is not the only factor that determines the prognosis or risk of the illness, and not all higher stage patients actually have high risk disease from a biologic standpoint. CLL carries some very unique prognostic or predictive factors that are not seen in other forms of lymphoma. One of these is the presence or absence of certain specific genetic abnormalities in the tumor cells, which does have some significance in terms of selection of therapy and does predict for likelihood of time to need therapy as well as likely duration of survival from the illness. Another difference is that in normal practice (i.e., outside of a clinical trial) the staging system for CLL relies less on the use of CT scans/PET scans and even potentially bone marrow biopsies to determine staging and remission status since the visibility of cells in the blood and very superficial areas of common lymph node enlargement mean that the simple determination of blood counts and performance of a physical exam are generally felt to be sufficient for determining stage and subsequent response to treatment.

Another way that CLL is somewhat unique from other types of lymphoma is in the presence of immune phenomena. Abnormalities in the immune system of patients with CLL may sometimes lead to the destruction of red cells causing anemia (autoimmune hemolytic anemia), or platelets (immune thrombocytopenia). Very rarely the patient's immune system may suppress red cell production completely or nearly completely (pure red cell aplasia). These are often treated with immune suppressive medicines to decrease the patient's immune system's activity against those cells. Finally either because of features of the illness itself or as a result of treatments used to treat CLL, patients with CLL appear somewhat more likely to develop viral or bacterial infections. If these infections are severe (e.g., requiring hospitalization for treatment) your physician may recommend monthly infusions of **intravenous immune globulin (IVIG)** to reduce the risk of subsequent infections.

General management of **indolent lymphomas** is discussed in Question 51 on page 109. A discussion of therapies specific to CLL/SLL is included in that section

21. What is lymphoplasmacytic lymphoma (Waldenstrom's macroglobulinemia)?

Lymphoplasmacytic lymphoma/Waldenstrom's macroglobulinemia (LPL/WM) is a disorder characterized by the excessive production of a specific type of antibody, **immunoglobulin M (IgM),** by the cells of a particular type of indolent lymphoma called LPL. The diagnosis is made by finding significant involvement of the bone marrow by the lymphoma cells along with a significantly elevated level of an abnormal IgM in the blood. Lymph nodes and spleen may be involved. There is another disorder called immunoglobulin M-monoclonal gammopathy of undetermined significance (IgM MGUS), in which there is a smaller degree of involvement of the bone marrow and a lower amount of the abnormal IgM in the blood. People with IgM MGUS need to be monitored but do not need any treatment. These people have a higher incidence of subsequently developing LPL/WM.

Intravenous immunoglobulin (IVIG)

A collection of pooled immunoglobulin G, obtained from many donors

Indolent lymphomas

A group of lymphomas that are generally slow growing and are usually treated only if causing important symptoms or signs of organ damage.

Waldenstrom's macroglobulinemia (WM)

A type of lymphoma that produces too much IgM and can be associated with an increased viscosity.

Immunoglobulin M (IgM)

One of the five different types of antibodies that are part of the immune system.

The lymphoma cells are mainly found in the bone marrow and lymph nodes. LPL/WM mainly affects older individuals, although occasional cases occur in younger people. It is a rare disorder, occurring more commonly in males than females.

There appears to be a slightly higher incidence of LPL/WM in people with hepatitis C infection, and it is likely that there are some as-yet unknown genetic factors, as there is also a slightly higher incidence in first-degree relatives. Otherwise, no cause is known.

Many patients have no symptoms at all at the time of diagnosis. Fatigue and a general sense of feeling unwell or malaise are often the only symptoms noticed. Anemia may be present. On physical examination, the patient may be pale as a result of the anemia. There may also be enlarged lymph nodes that can be felt or an enlarged liver or spleen.

The presence of an elevated IgM level is confirmed by blood tests. IgM is an antibody normally found in the blood, where it has a role in protecting and fighting against infection. However, when too much of one type of IgM is produced, the excess can be detected by special blood tests (serum protein electrophoresis and immunofixation). These abnormal tests may sometimes be the first clue to the presence of this type of lymphoma.

In addition to problems related to the presence of the lymphoma itself, the excessive IgM protein can also cause its own set of problems. This particular immunoglobulin molecule joins up with four other molecules of the same type to circulate in the blood as a very large molecule. The five molecules joined together form a very large protein that, when present in excessive amounts, can cause the blood to become too thick, resulting in a **hyperviscosity** syndrome. The hyperviscosity syndrome is associated with sluggish blood flow and can result in dizziness, tiredness, headache, vision changes, confusion, and sometimes bleeding. Patients with hyperviscosity syndrome may also have signs and symptoms of heart failure. When suspected, a test known as a serum viscosity can be performed to see if the circulating protein in the plasma is causing the symptoms in question. The development of the hyperviscosity syndrome indicates the need for fairly urgent **plasmapheresis**. Plasmapheresis can decrease the amount of IgM in the serum relatively quickly, resulting in resolution of the signs and symptoms of hyperviscosity. However definitive treatment for the lymphoma must also be started at that point since plasmapheresis only removes existing IgM in the serum but does not decrease its production by the lymphoma cells. This is the job of the subsequent chemotherapy or **immunotherapy**. It is important to understand that a high serum viscosity test result in the absence of any symptoms is not an indication by itself that the hyperviscosity syndrome is present.

The IgM can cause problems by attaching to normal body components such as the lining of nerves or other tissues or proteins in the blood. In the case of nerves, this can cause **peripheral neuropathy** (numbness, tingling and pain in the fingers and toes, and, occasionally, weakness). Neuropathy affects approximately 20% of patients with WM/LPL. The IgM protein can also be associated with **Raynaud's syndrome**, a disorder in which the hands get painful and the fingers change from white to blue and then to red when exposed to the cold. Bleeding problems can also be due to the protein attaching to platelets or other blood proteins that are important for preventing bleeding.

Hyperviscosity

A condition in which the blood is too thick.

Plasmapheresis

A treatment that consists of removing plasma.

Immunotherapy

Treatment aimed at controlling the immune system.

Peripheral neuropathy

A condition caused by damage to the nerves in the arms or legs.

Raynaud's syndrome

A disorder associated with pain and a change in blood flow and color in the fingers.

DIAGNOSIS AND CLASSIFICATION OF LYMPHOMA

The treatment of this type of lymphoma is similar to that of the other types of indolent lymphomas, with the exception of the previously mentioned problem of hyperviscosity. This lymphoma, like the others in this group, is not considered to be curable with conventional types of chemotherapy. A common approach, with the intent of maintaining well-being and minimizing the risks of side effects, is to only treat when the lymphoma is causing either problems related to significant falls in the blood counts or bothersome symptoms such as fever, sweats, weight loss, and painful or bothersome neuropathy. **Antibody therapy** with monoclonal antibodies, chemotherapy, or a combination of these treatments are all reasonable options. Following monoclonal antibodies, responses may continue to improve over many months. Initially, the IgM level may actually go up in the early period following this therapy, giving the appearance that the treatment has not worked, but this may be misleading. A flare reaction where the IgM level rises has been seen following monoclonal antibody therapy and hyperviscosity can develop as a result. A course of plasmapheresis may be needed for a short period of time in some patients.

Chemotherapy agents that are effective include chlorambucil and cyclophosphamide, and both of these can be taken in pill form. These treatments are used less frequently today, as there are more effective and better-tolerated treatments available. However, they can still be a very good choice, especially in older people who wish for less aggressive therapies. Fludarabine and the related drugs cladribine and pentostatin are also very effective drugs. The regimen known as CHOP (see Question 51 on page 109) in conjunction with a monoclonal antibody such as rituximab is an effective treatment. Monoclonal antibodies on their own can be effective therapy but should be used with caution in patients with high IgM

Antibody therapy

The use of antibodies to treat cancer.

levels as the levels have been reported to temporarily increase after monoclonal therapy. Also since some biologic features and behaviors of this illness overlap with an illness known as multiple myeloma, many of the agents used for multiple myeloma (e.g., thalidomide, bortezomib) are also useful for treating this illness. A better understanding of the abnormal molecular pathways that are disturbed within lymphoma cells has led to the development of more targeted agents that are being tested in lymphomas such as this. One such example is ibrutinib, an agent which blocks an enzyme known as a Bruton's tyrosine kinase which is abnormally active in many types of lymphomas, leading to arrest of growth of the lymphoma cells. This agent is now approved for use in the USA for mantle cell lymphoma and CLL (see Questions 20 and 26 on pages 50 and 68) that have recurred or are not responsive to initial therapies.

More aggressive treatments may be considered for younger people, especially for those who have disease that has been difficult to control with standard options. High-dose chemotherapy or chemoradiotherapy with **autologous stem cell transplant** can be associated with more durable responses in some patients; however, it is important to realize that this is not a cure. Even more investigational is an allogeneic transplant. There is some evidence that a graft-versus-LPL/WM effect occurs, and this treatment has curative potential. Ideally, it should be performed in the setting of a clinical trial.

As previously mentioned plasmapheresis is an option when it is necessary to remove the excess IgM quickly, effectively thinning the blood, for the short term. For longer-term control, a course of monoclonal antibody therapy and/or chemotherapy may also be helpful to decrease the protein (IgM) production.

Autologous stem cell transplant

A transplant in which one is one's own bone marrow stem cell donor.

More aggressive treatments may be considered for younger people, especially for those who have disease that has been difficult to control with standard options.

To perform plasmapheresis, two intravenous needles are placed into your arms. One intravenous needle delivers your blood to the plasmapheresis machine. The other returns the blood back to your body. In the machine, the IgM is separated from the rest of your blood, which is then returned to your body.

22. What is follicular lymphoma—grade 1–2?

Grade 1–2 follicular lymphoma is the second most common type of non-Hodgkin lymphoma, accounting for approximately 10–20% of all cases. This type of lymphoma is determined by the number of large cells present among the small lymphocytes (small cleaved cells) that make up the bulk of the lymphoma cells. The older WHO classification split this lymphoma into grade 1 and grade 2, based on the number of large lymphocytes present in the biopsy specimen. Because the separation of grade 1 and grade 2 was inconsistent between pathologists and no clear difference in prognosis between the groups was shown, the newer classification combined them together as grade 1–2. More is understood about the abnormalities that occur in the lymphocytes leading to this type of lymphoma than in many other lymphomas. A hallmark of this type of lymphoma is the presence of too much of a protein called Bcl-2. A gene called bcl-2 produces this protein, and the excess Bcl-2 allows the lymphocyte to live longer than is normal. Because the abnormal lymphocytes fail to die, which happens during normal cell turnover, too many lymphocytes accumulate, eventually forming lymph node tumors. The reason for the overproduction of Bcl-2 is also understood. All humans have 23 pairs of chromosomes—46 chromosomes in all—that contain many, many genes. The genes are made up of **deoxyribonucleic acid (DNA)**, and each contains the fundamental information necessary for the manufacture of a protein. The process responsible for making a protein from the message contained in a gene is normally regulated very closely in order to prevent too much of a protein being produced. Sometimes genes can get moved from one chromosome to another; such an event is called **translocation**. In the **follicular lymphomas**, the gene for the production of the Bcl-2 protein gets moved from chromosome 18 to chromosome 14. On chromosome 14, bcl-2 is placed next to another gene that gives it instructions to keep producing the Bcl-2 protein. As mentioned previously, the Bcl-2 protein prevents the lymphocyte from dying at the right time. Normal lymphocytes are programmed to die at the end of their normal life span. This built-in death program is called **apoptosis** (programmed cell death) and is essentially a cell suicide program. If this process is blocked (e.g., by having too much Bcl-2), lymphocytes accumulate, and lymphoma may result. Many chemotherapy drugs that are useful in lymphoma act by causing lymphocytes to undergo programmed cell death, but when too much Bcl-2 is present, the lymphoma can be more resistant to chemotherapy. Clinical trials evaluating compounds that could be given to patients to specifically block the Bcl-2 protein from performing its normal function are ongoing. The hope is that this will then allow cells to die normally and also to respond better to chemotherapy. It appears that monoclonal antibodies act partly through activation of cell death pathways. In October 2002, the Nobel Prize for medicine was awarded to researchers who discovered the basics of this important cell suicide program.

The average age at which this type of lymphoma occurs is 55 to 60 years. Most types of lymphoma occur in equal frequency in males and females, although some

Deoxyribonucleic acid (DNA)

The material that carries the genetic code for each organism or person.

Translocation

An abnormality of certain chromosomes seen in some cancer cells.

Follicular lymphomas

Lymphomas composed of lymphocytes organized into round structures.

Apoptosis

A process by which normal cells die. Some cancer cells do not die, and a failure of cells to undergo apoptosis can contribute to the growth of cancer. It is often referred to as "programmed cell death."

DIAGNOSIS AND CLASSIFICATION OF LYMPHOMA

subtypes of lymphoma are more common in one gender (e.g., mantle cell lymphoma is much more common in males). Approximately half of the patients with stage IV lymphoma will have B symptoms (fevers, night sweats, and weight loss), but the symptoms occur much less frequently in patients with stage I to stage III disease.

Often, the first noticeable sign is the presence of a new painless lump in the neck or groin that may have been present for several weeks or months. With indolent lymphomas such as follicular lymphoma grade 1-2 the size of the lymph node may vary in size over time, maybe even getting smaller (waxing and waning). If a follicular lymphoma is expected by the history, it is generally preferable for the surgeon to remove the entire lymph node (an excisional biopsy) for examination. The pathologist will be more likely to be sure of the diagnosis if more tissue is available to examine. This is because part of the diagnosis of follicular lymphoma is made on the basis of the architectural appearance (i.e., the distribution) of the malignant cells within the node. Since the cells have a tendency to grow in a focal (follicular) or nodular pattern, it is important for the pathologist to be able to see these **follicles** or nodules within the biopsy material. In a small biopsy there may not be a large enough sample to be able to see this characteristic. and a subsequent excisional biopsy may be needed.

Follicles

Round structures containing lymphocytes.

In some cases, the only enlarged lymph nodes may not be easy to biopsy. Examples include lymph nodes deep inside the chest, between the lungs, or inside the abdomen. In these cases, needle aspirations or core needle biopsies may be all that are possible. A laparoscopic biopsy (keyhole surgery) can sometimes be performed to obtain a larger piece of the lymph node.

You will be referred to a **hematologist/oncologist** after a diagnosis is made. At that point, staging tests are performed, and decisions about treatment are discussed.

23. What is marginal zone lymphoma?

Marginal zone lymphoma is an indolent type of lymphoma that arises from the marginal zone of lymph node follicles. They arise either in lymph nodes (nodal marginal zone lymphoma), the spleen (splenic marginal zone lymphoma), or in association with mucous membrane tissues (the mucosa-associated lymphoid tissue or **MALT lymphomas**). They are generally slow growing and tend to occur in older individuals. The name *marginal* comes from the area in the lymph node surrounding the follicle that is most abnormal when the lymph node is examined under the microscope. This type of lymphoma can also occasionally occur in areas such as the lung or breast without being found elsewhere in the body.

Nodal marginal zone lymphoma is rare, accounting for only approximately 2% of all lymphoma cases. At diagnosis there is generally no involvement of the spleen or other sites outside of lymph nodes, apart from the bone marrow in this type of lymphoma. Patients will often have stage III or IV disease at the time of diagnosis, as is common with most of the indolent lymphomas. B symptoms are uncommon, and, most frequently the lymph nodes may be found by the patient or his/her physician during a routine medical exam. Similar to other indolent lymphomas, this type of lymphoma is generally considered to be incurable but is controllable, and patients often can remain well and without symptoms for long periods of time. If treatment is required at some point in time, options include monoclonal antibodies alone or in combination with chemotherapy.

Hematologist/ oncologist

A physician specializing in the treatment of blood disorders and cancer.

MALT lymphomas

A type of lymphoma that tends to involve lymph glands present in the mucosa (the lining of the gut or other organs).

Splenic marginal zone lymphoma is also a rare type of lymphoma, accounting for less than 1% of all lymphoma cases. The spleen is often found to be very large, and it is common to find lymphoma cells circulating in the bone marrow and blood, as well as in lymph nodes. In the circulation, the circulating lymphocytes often appear to have strands growing out and are called villous lymphocytes. This type of lymphoma appears to occur more frequently in people who are infected with the hepatitis C virus, especially in Mediterranean countries and Japan. There are reports that some cases may regress/go into remission through the treatment of hepatitis C. This tends to be an indolent-behaving lymphoma. Symptoms are often due to the enlarged spleen, which, when very enlarged, takes up a lot of space within the abdomen and can lead to abdominal discomfort; early satiety, which is the sensation of being full after eating only a small amount of food; and heartburn. The enlarged spleen can also hide or soak up (sequester) normal circulating blood cells like a sponge, so the blood counts can fall. Another cause for the low blood counts is bone marrow involvement by the lymphoma. The diagnosis of splenic marginal zone lymphoma is often made by examination of the bone marrow or by performing flow cytometry on the circulating blood. These tests are easier than removing the spleen, which is another way of making the diagnosis. Consideration may be given to removing the spleen if the diagnosis is still not certain from the other tests, or occasionally if other therapies have not worked. Removing the spleen can also improve the blood counts since it removes the source that is sequestering the circulating cells, and will relieve the sensation of abdominal fullness that patients often experience symptoms associated with its presence in the abdomen. However the spleen is part of the immune system and removing it increases slightly the chance of developing certain types of bacterial infection (*Streptococcus Pneumoniae, Neisseria Meningiditis,* and *Hemophilus Influenzae*). Very rarely patients who lack a spleen can develop rapid life-threatening bloodstream infections from these bacteria, and this needs to be considered as the decision to consider removing the spleen is being made. Vaccines against these bacteria are available and should be given prior to a planned splenectomy if possible. If other therapy is needed or if taking out the spleen is not an option, monoclonal antibodies can be very effective by themselves or when combined with other forms of chemotherapy.

MALT lymphomas occur in areas outside of lymph nodes. They generally affect the mucosa (lining) of the gut, **salivary glands**, tissues surrounding the eye (orbital or ocular), lung, thyroid, breast, bladder, or kidney. They are an uncommon type of indolent lymphoma. This subtype of lymphoma is often localized (confined to one area) at the time of diagnosis. Bone marrow involvement is unusual. These lymphomas tend to be slow growing and are more common in people with an autoimmune disorder affecting the area where there has been chronic inflammation, related to the autoimmune disorder. For example MALT lymphoma involving the salivary gland occurs more frequently in people with Sjögren's syndrome, and the thyroid form of this lymphoma occurs more frequently in people with **Hashimoto's thyroiditis**. These are autoimmune disorders in which the body forms antibodies that attack the salivary glands or thyroid gland. Interestingly, in cases of MALT lymphomas, the site of involvement (e.g., stomach, lung) does not normally have much or any developed lymphoid tissue present at that site. It is generally felt that the lymphocytes accumulate at the site in question because of signals sent by an infectious or

Salivary glands

The gland that produces saliva.

Hashimoto's thyroiditis

A type of inflammation of the thyroid due to abnormal recognition of the thyroid gland as foreign.

inflammatory process, eventually leading to the development of the lymphoma. The best example of this is the development of gastric MALT lymphomas because of the presence of *Helicobacter pylori* in the stomach, described here.

Gastric MALT or MALT lymphoma involving the stomach is the most common form of MALT lymphoma. It is associated with an infection by a bacterium called *Helicobacter pylori* in most cases. It appears that the presence of inflammation caused by the bacteria in the stomach leads to accumulation of the lymphocytes that eventually lead to a lymphoma. The diagnosis is usually made by performing an upper gastrointestinal **endoscopy** with biopsies of areas appearing to be abnormal. Patients may complain of upper abdominal discomfort or bloating, nausea, or dyspepsia. Giving antibiotics to patients with both stomach lymphoma and this infection has resulted in remission, even without chemotherapy, in approximately three-quarters of patients. A number of tests can be done to evaluate for the presence of the *Helicobacter pylori* bacteria. These include special stains of the biopsy by the pathologist, a urea breath test, or a blood test to evaluate for antibodies to the bacteria. More than one test should be done before concluding that the lymphoma is not associated with the bacteria and deciding that treatment with antibiotics will not be helpful. Other infectious agents, including hepatitis C and *Borrelia burgdorferi*, the agent that causes Lyme disease, have also been implicated in the development of a similar lymphoma at other sites.

After diagnosis, patients with gastric MALT need to undergo staging, as with all other types of lymphoma. If the lymphoma is present only within the stomach and the test for *Helicobacter pylori* is positive, a course of

Endoscopy

A procedure to examine the gut with a fiber optic light.

antibiotics along with an acid-blocking medicine is the usual treatment. After antibiotic treatment, it may take a long time (a year or more) for the lymphoma to completely disappear, and repeat endoscopies periodically throughout the year are necessary to ensure that the lymphoma is continuing to respond. If the lymphoma is not associated with the *Helicobacter pylori* bacteria, low-dose radiation can provide excellent control. If there is involvement in areas outside the stomach, either monoclonal antibodies alone or given with a chemotherapy regimen will usually be appropriate. Surgery is generally not necessary. Very rarely cases of DLBCL localized to the stomach have been associated with *Helicobacter pylori*. It is possible that these cases may have represented unrecognized gastric MALT lymphomas that transformed to a higher-grade lymphoma. Although DLBCL is nearly always treated with aggressive chemotherapy regimens, cases associated with *Helicobacter pylori* have been reported to respond to antibiotic therapy directed against this organism. The use of antibiotic therapy in this instance should only be considered very carefully since monitoring of response to therapy since this type of lymphoma can behave in a very aggressive fashion.

MALT lymphomas affecting other areas of the body tend to behave in a very indolent or low-grade fashion. They can involve the thyroid gland, conjunctival tissue in the eye, the parotid gland, skin, breast tissue, and areas of the gut other than the stomach. Similar to *Helicobacter pylori* and gastric MALT, other infections have been reported in a few cases of MALT lymphoma occurring at other sites, although these associations are much less consistent than they are for *Helicobacter pylori* and gastric MALT lymphoma. They include *Borrelia burgdorferi* in MALT lymphomas affecting the skin, *Campylobacter jejuni* in lymphomas affecting the bowel, and *Chlamydia*

*Local irradia-
tion can be a
very effective
treatment in
many cases
of MALT
lymphoma,
providing
long-term
complete con-
trol or cure in
most patients.*

trachomatis in conjunctival MALT lymphomas. For these non-gastric types of marginal zone lymphoma, if there is localized involvement, surgical removal may be recommended, and radiation may also be an option. Local irradiation can be a very effective treatment in many cases of MALT lymphoma, providing long-term complete control or cure in most patients. As is the case with many types of lymphoma, if there is involvement of more than one site, a monoclonal antibody with or without chemotherapy may be recommended.

24. What is follicular grade 3 non-Hodgkin lymphoma?

Follicular lymphomas are currently divided into two groups. They are grade 1–2 and grade 3. Grade 3 is also divided into grade 3A and grade 3B, based on the pathologist's evaluation of the number of larger cells present in the biopsy. Follicular grade 1–2 lymphomas are generally considered to be indolent lymphomas, whereas grade 3 is considered to be an aggressive lymphoma. In reality, grade 3A may behave more like the indolent lymphomas and grade 3B more like the aggressive lymphomas. Unfortunately, this situation is more complicated, as the ability of most pathologists to distinguish between grade 3A and 3B is often not very good. This is based on studies showing that when the same biopsy is looked at by different pathologists, there is frequent disagreement on the grade.

Grade 3 lymphomas are the least common of the follicular lymphomas. Staging of these lymphomas is the same as for other types of non-Hodgkin lymphoma, and the treatment is similar to that of either other indolent follicular non-Hodgkin lymphomas or DLBCLs (see

Question 25 on page 67), depending on the specific grade and patient-related features.

In practice, because the difference between grade 3A and 3B is difficult to determine, most patients are just classified as having grade 3 lymphoma. The treatment is most commonly chemotherapy with the CHOP (H = Adriamycin [Hydroxydaunorubicin] O = vincristine [Oncovin] P = predisone) regimen (see Question 51 on page 109) combined with a monoclonal antibody. The goal of treatment is a cure. The likelihood of a cure, however, may be lower than that seen with diffuse large B-cell lymphoma-not otherwise specified (DLBCL-NOS) and the other aggressive lymphomas.

25. What are diffuse large B-cell lymphoma-not otherwise specified (DLBCL-NOS) and the other types of aggressive lymphoma?

DLBCL-NOS is the most common type of lymphoma. It accounts for approximately 30–40% of all lymphoma cases. DLBCL-NOS occurs mostly in adults of middle age and older but is also not uncommon in younger individuals. The average age at which patients develop this type of lymphoma is 60 years. Many cases are curable with chemotherapy combined with a monoclonal antibody, but if they are not treated, the lymphoma usually grows rapidly and can result in death within six months to a year. Most of these lymphomas arise from B-lymphocytes, but 25% arise from T cells. T-cell lymphomas are generally more resistant to treatment than B-cell lymphomas.

One-third of these lymphomas are localized when first diagnosed. The occurrence of the lymphoma at sites other than the lymph nodes, including the bone marrow, gut, lungs, kidneys, and liver, is not uncommon.

Often, the first symptom noted may be a rapidly growing lump that is generally painless, but tenderness may be noted because the capsule of the lymph node gets stretched rapidly. Initially, patients may be observed or given antibiotics to treat a suspected infection, as this is a more likely cause of lymph node swelling. If the lymph node does not return to normal (or continues to grow) over a few weeks with or without antibiotics, a lymph node biopsy should be obtained. Abdominal pain or discomfort, cough, shortness of breath, or a sensation of fullness in the chest or neck may also be the first abnormality noted. Fevers and night sweats may occur, and weight loss may also be noted (these are the B symptoms).

A number of different lymphomas are classified in the aggressive lymphoma group. Previously, they had been listed together with DLBCL but now they have been separated. They are listed in **Table 7** but aside from Burkitt lymphoma, they are not discussed in detail in this book, as they are relatively infrequent. Burkitt lymphoma and related disorders are generally described as highly aggressive.

26. What is mantle cell lymphoma?

Mantle cell lymphoma accounts for approximately 5–7% of all lymphomas. Men are affected approximately four times as often as women. Mantle cell lymphoma has traditionally been included with the indolent lymphomas

Table 7 Aggressive B-cell lymphomas in the WHO Classification (2008)

Diffuse large B-cell lymphoma, not otherwise specified

    Primary DLBCL of the CNS

    Primary cutaneous DLBCL, leg type

    T cell/histiocyte rich large B-cell lymphoma

    EBV+ DLBCL of the elderly

DLBCL associated with chronic inflammation

Primary mediastinal (thymic) large B-cell lymphoma

Intravascular large B-cell lymphoma ALK+ large B-cell lymphoma

Plasmablastic lymphoma

Primary effusion lymphoma

Large B-cell lymphoma arising in HHV-8–associated multicentric Castleman Disease

Highly Aggressive B-cell lymphomas

Burkitt lymphoma

B-cell lymphoma, unclassifiable, with features intermediate between diffuse large B-cell lymphoma and Burkitt lymphoma

B-cell lymphoma, unclassifiable, with features intermediate between diffuse large B-cell lymphoma and classical Hodgkin lymphoma

Modified from: The 2008 WHO classification of lymphomas: implications for clinical practice and translational research Elaine S. Jaffe Hematopathology Section, Laboratory of Pathology, Center for Cancer Research, National Cancer Institute, National Institutes of Health, Bethesda, MD ASH Education Book January 1, 2009 vol. 2009 no. 1 523-531

(because it is generally considered incurable), although clinically it demonstrates a wide range of behaviors and growth rates. Many physicians will treat it with regimens used for aggressive and even highly aggressive lymphoma as it tends to grow faster than other indolent lymphomas, and the overall survival appears to be shorter. As a result, most patients will need treatment when the diagnosis is first made, although in some cases without rapidly growing masses, this lymphoma may be watched without initial therapy.

Mantle cell lymphoma occurs mostly in older adults. Patients often have enlarged lymph nodes at many sites, often with a large liver and spleen because of lymphoma involvement.

Mantle cell lymphoma occurs mostly in older adults. Patients often have enlarged lymph nodes at many sites, often with a large liver and spleen because of lymphoma involvement. The bone marrow is also commonly involved. Lymphoma cells may also be found in the bloodstream in up to 50% of patients. Another common site is the gut, especially the colon. Sometimes an abnormality found in the gut at the time of endoscopy may lead to the diagnosis of mantle cell lymphoma. If a diagnosis of mantle cell lymphoma has been made, even if there are no gastrointestinal symptoms, your physician may want you to undergo endoscopy.

Like most other types of lymphoma, the cause of mantle cell lymphoma is unknown. As is the case with overproduction of Bcl-2 in the follicular lymphomas, the lymphoma cells in this disorder overproduce a protein called Bcl-1, which causes the abnormal lymphocytes to grow faster and accumulate. Bcl-1 is also known as cyclin D1. The abnormal production of Bcl-1 is the result of a chromosomal translocation, t(11:14), where some genes on one chromosome move to another chromosome. The abnormal lymphocytes also express CD5, a protein, on their surfaces. Mantle cell lymphoma is a B-cell lymphoma, and CD5 is not normally present on B cells (though it is normally present on some T cells). CD5 is also seen in another B-cell leukemia/lymphoma, CLL/SLL, and it is important to distinguish between these two types, as the management is different. One helpful distinguishing feature is CD23, a protein that is usually present on the surface of the lymphoma cells in CLL/SLL but absent from the surface of the lymphocytes in mantle cell lymphoma.

Patients will often have disease at multiple sites at the diagnosis, often being stage III or IV. B symptoms, including fevers, night sweats, and weight loss, are not uncommon.

Once the diagnosis is made and staging has been completed, treatment is usually initiated. As with the follicular lymphomas, most patients respond well initially to treatment, sometimes even achieving a complete response (disappearance of all visible evidence of disease); however, on average, the time before the disease comes back is shorter than it is with the follicular lymphomas.

The treatment of indolent lymphomas is discussed in Question 51 on page 109. Although mantle cell lymphoma has features that overlap with indolent and aggressive lymphomas, it is included in the section on indolent lymphoma. Some very intensive treatments including blood transplantation may help to improve long term-outcomes in this group of lymphomas.

27. What is Burkitt lymphoma?

Burkitt lymphoma is a very rapidly growing lymphoma but is curable in a high percentage of people. It is considered to be a highly aggressive B-cell lymphoma. Both Burkitt and Burkitt-like lymphomas have been described in previous classifications and with the most recent update to the WHO classification, most cases of Burkitt-like lymphoma would now be classified as "B-cell lymphoma, unclassifiable, with features intermediate between diffuse large B-cell lymphoma and Burkitt lymphoma" (B-UNC/BL/DLBCL). Both types behave similarly and as a result of more similarities than differences, the distinction between them is becoming less significant; Burkitt lymphomas occur

Burkitt lymphoma

A very rapidly growing and aggressive type of lymphoma.

predominantly in children whereas B-UNC/BL/ DLBC lymphoma affects older adults.

Burkitt lymphoma was named for Denis Burkitt, an Irish surgeon who, while working in East Africa, noticed large tumors occurring in the jaws of children. He reported this disease in 1958.

The following three types of Burkitt lymphoma are recognized:

1. Endemic Burkitt lymphoma
2. **Sporadic Burkitt** lymphoma
3. Immunodeficiency-associated Burkitt lymphoma

Sporadic Burkitt

The form of Burkitt lymphoma that occurs in the United States.

Endemic Burkitt lymphoma occurs mainly in equatorial Africa. It affects approximately 1 in 10,000 children and accounts for 50% of cancers seen in children in this part of the world. It most commonly presents as a tumor of the jaw or face and typically affects males between the ages of 4 and 7. This lymphoma does not occur in adults. It is usually a very rapidly growing tumor and can affect the upper or lower jaw or even both at the same time. Involvement of lymph nodes or bone marrow is uncommon. Involvement of the nervous system occurs more commonly than in the non-African type. This type of lymphoma is almost always associated with the EBV.

Sporadic Burkitt lymphoma in the US affects 1 in 400,000 children, accounting for approximately one-third of all of lymphomas seen in children. It also affects adults. It affects males more commonly than females, and tumors involving the abdomen or bowel are most common. Gastrointestinal complaints are frequently present in patients with this type of lymphoma. They include nausea, vomiting, abdominal pain; symptoms related to bowel involvement/obstruction. Back pain may also occur, and any leg weakness or sensation disturbance should raise concern for a mass pressing on the spinal cord, which is a medical emergency. Frequently, the bowel, pancreas, kidneys, and surrounding lymph nodes are involved.

Involvement of the ovaries is common in females. Bone marrow involvement, which implies a poorer prognosis and also makes **central nervous system (CNS)** involvement more likely, is unusual, occurring in 20% of patients. B symptoms do not occur frequently with this type of lymphoma. EBV infection is much less common in this type of Burkitt lymphoma. Another way for this type of lymphoma to present is with bone marrow and blood involvement.

Central nervous system (CNS)

The brain and spinal cord.

Immunodeficiency-associated Burkitt lymphoma occurs in patients with HIV infection or AIDS, or in people who are immunosuppressed for other reasons. This can occur in solid organ transplant recipients for whom lifelong continuation of immunosuppressive therapy is required. In most cases, there is involvement of lymph nodes or bone marrow.

When the pathologist examines these lymphomas under the microscope, often sheets of monotonous medium sized cells are present. A characteristic finding under the microscope is described as the "starry sky appearance" that is created by the death of some of the rapidly growing cells that are subsequently taken up by resident macrophages in the lymph node.

The cause of these lymphomas remains unknown, but EBV is variably involved as previously described.

They occur more frequently in people with depressed immune systems, especially those infected with HIV. These associations suggest some role for an abnormality of the immune system in allowing these lymphomas to develop. An abnormality is also seen at the genetic level, involving the lymphocytes of most patients with these lymphomas. A protein called c-Myc is overproduced because the gene that controls the production of this protein gets moved to a different chromosome, where its production is continuously turned on. Too much of the protein drives the abnormal cell growth. This is typically a translocation between chromosomes 8 and 14, commonly written as t(8;14), and occurs in all three types of Burkitt lymphoma.

28. What is lymphoblastic lymphoma?

Lymphoblastic lymphoma, another of the high-grade, very aggressive lymphomas, is an uncommon lymphoma. It occurs more frequently in children and adolescents than in adults, and accounts for one-third of all lymphomas occurring in children but less than 5% of adult lymphomas. Most of these lymphomas (80%) are T-cell lymphomas, whereas the remainder are B-cell lymphomas. The pathologist is able to distinguish this type of lymphoma with a microscope. The lymphocytes appear very immature and can be stained for a particular enzyme, terminal deoxynucleotidyl transferase, which is not commonly seen with other types of lymphoma. This lymphoma has many features in common with **acute lymphoblastic leukemia** and in the latest WHO classification, it is listed either under B lymphoblastic leukemia/lymphoma or T-cell lymphoblastic leukemia/lymphoma.

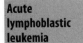

Acute lymphoblastic leukemia

A fast-growing type of leukemia.

Lymphoblastic lymphoma occurs mostly in males and, when seen in adults, usually occurs between the ages of 20 and 30. It presents most frequently with a mass in the anterior mediastinum, the space between the front of the lungs and the chest wall. This can be associated with fluid collection around the heart (pericardial effusion) or around the lungs (pleural effusion). Often, enlarged lymph nodes also occur in the neck or armpits. If the chest mass grows very quickly, it can cause pressure on the **trachea** (windpipe) or blood vessels. When this occurs, patients may complain of chest pain, shortness of breath, a choking sensation, headaches, or problems with vision. When the flow of blood returning to the heart is diminished by a large tumor mass, a superior vena cava syndrome may occur. This is a relative medical emergency, and, if a rapidly growing lymphoma causes these symptoms, an urgent biopsy should be followed by treatment fairly immediately.

Trachea
The windpipe.

29. What are immunodeficiency-associated lymphoproliferative disorders (including HIV-, post-transplant –, and methotrexate-associated lymphoma)?

A number of primary immunodeficiencies are associated with abnormal T-cell number and function. This creates a situation that allows for increased susceptibility to infections. EBV infection is more likely to occur and is associated with an increased risk of developing lymphoma. The same virus causes infectious mononucleosis. The primary immunodeficiencies associated with an increased risk of lymphoma are the Wiskott-Aldrich syndrome, severe combined immunodeficiency (SCID), and common variable immunodeficiency (CVID). Wiskott-Aldrich syndrome is a genetic abnormality characterized by immunodeficiency, decreased and abnormal platelets with a bleeding tendency, and eczema. SCID is due to genetic abnormalities that affect normal immune responses. CVID refers to a group of illnesses characterized by low immune globulin levels and often functional abnormalities in the immune response to various infections. Individuals with CVID generally have recurring infections beginning after two years of age and generally require life-long infusions of IVIG on a monthly basis or so.

HIV-Associated Lymphoma

The incidence of a number of different types of lymphomas is increased in individuals with the HIV infection. The higher viral loads and lower CD4+ blood counts contribute to the risk of developing lymphoma. The risk of developing lymphoma has decreased since the introduction of HAART, which results in higher CD4+ counts. Lymphomas seen in individuals with HIV are often associated with the EBV or the Kaposi's sarcoma herpesvirus, which is also known as HHV8. These viruses seem to be at least partly responsible for the development of the lymphoma. These virus infections occur more commonly with the immune suppression caused by HIV. The lymphomas seen more commonly in HIV infected individuals include Burkitt lymphoma and DLBCL. There is also appears to be an increased incidence of Hodgkin lymphoma.

PEL is a rare lymphoma that generally occurs in the setting of HIV infection. PEL is virtually always associated with Kaposi's sarcoma herpesvirus, and, instead of involving lymph nodes or organs, fluid collections or effusions appear in the pleural cavity (the lining around the lungs) or the peritoneal cavity (the lining around the abdominal organs), resulting in the development of ascites. It is often difficult to make the diagnosis in such cases, as lymphoma often will not be suspected. Another type of lymphoma that can appear similar to PEL occurs in patients infected with the hepatitis C virus. In addition to normal staging tests, patients with lymphoma who are HIV-positive will often require a lumbar puncture to evaluate the cerebrospinal fluid (CSF) for evidence of involvement of the nervous system.

CNS lymphoma is more common in these patients. It can be either primary or secondary CNS lymphoma. **Intrathecal** chemotherapy is often administered at the time the first lumbar puncture is done. Unless the pathologist sees lymphoma cells, the intrathecal chemotherapy is given for prophylaxis. If there is any concern about primary CNS lymphoma, a magnetic resonance imaging (MRI) scan is more sensitive than a CT scan for ruling out other lesions that may occur in HIV-positive individuals. A brain biopsy may be necessary in this situation.

Plasmablastic lymphoma is always associated with the HHV8 virus in HIV infected individuals. These lymphomas can present as masses occurring in the mouth and sinuses or affecting mucosal sites in other areas.

Given that lymphomas diagnosed in the in the setting of immunodeficiency are often aggressive, symptoms can be severe at presentation or affected individuals can present with a fever-of-unknown origin. Often, areas outside of the lymph nodes can be involved at the time of diagnosis and may include the bone marrow, liver, gut, lungs and CNS. Individuals with CNS involvement

Intrathecal

The administration of a substance, often chemotherapy, into the fluid surrounding the spinal cord and brain.

Plasmablastic lymphoma

A rare type of lymphoma due to immature plasma cells.

may have no neurologic symptoms whatsoever, or may have headache, neck pain, back pain, motor or sensory changes, altered mental status, or cranial nerve abnormalities.

Post-Transplant Lymphomas

There is an increased risk of lymphoma both after solid organ transplants and bone marrow or stem cell transplants (when the marrow or stem cell donor is an individual other than the patient, i.e., an allogeneic donor). When it occurs, it is referred to as PTLD. It most frequently occurs after a lung or heart transplant and less often, after a kidney transplant. It can occur after any type of organ transplant and is related to the use of immune suppression which the organ recipient is required to take after the transplant. PTLD occurs less frequently after allogeneic peripheral blood stem cell or marrow transplants. This may be related in part to differences in immunosuppressive regimens for solid organ transplants compared to allogeneic marrow/peripheral blood stem cell transplants. Also patients receiving allogeneic marrow/peripheral blood cell transplants may not need to take immunosuppression for life. There are a number of different conditions included under the umbrella term PTLD. These range from a benign but abnormal lymph node enlargement that can be at one site or many sites throughout the body and can behave like infectious mononucleosis to a very rapidly growing, aggressive lymphoma that may involve the transplanted organ in addition to other parts of the body. In such cases, the lymph nodes may not be involved.

Most post-transplant lymphomas arise from B-lymphocytes and are associated with the Epstein-Barr virus (EBV), which stimulates B-lymphocytes to grow. It appears that people who have received a transplant and need to be kept on medication to suppress the immune system to prevent rejection of the transplanted organ are particularly vulnerable to EBV infection. The immune-suppressing medications primarily suppress T lymphocyte function, which normally keeps EBV in check. When T lymphocytes are not functioning properly, the lack of T-cell function may allow the EBV to reactivate. If EBV infection occurs for the first time or is reactivated in someone who was previously infected, a risk of developing lymphoma exists. Most of the adult population has been infected with EBV, which frequently does not cause illness but stays dormant in the body. Fortunately, the development of lymphoma only rarely occurs. It is estimated that 1% of kidney transplant recipients develop this type of lymphoma. The incidence is a little higher in heart and lung transplant recipients (possibly up to 6%). In bone marrow or **stem cell transplantation**, the risk of PTLD increases if T cells are removed from the graft. T cells are sometimes removed to try to prevent the complication of **graft-versus-host disease (GVHD)** (see Question 88 on page 184).

Treatment of this type of lymphoma is often quite different than for other lymphomas. The first step is to reduce the dose of the immune-suppressing antirejection drugs whenever possible. This is easier to do in patients with kidney and bone marrow transplants, but is much more complicated and difficult to do following a vital organ transplant, such as the heart or lung. Patients may respond simply to withdrawal of these antirejection drugs. If further treatment is needed, monoclonal antibodies are often given next. If even further therapy is needed for progression or relapse, chemotherapy along with monoclonal antibodies is given.

Stem cell transplantation

The procedure of replacing bone marrow stem cells to allow recovery of blood cells after high-dose chemotherapy.

Graft-versus-host disease (GVHD)

An illness caused by the donor's immune system recognizing and attacking tissues and organs of the patient.

Prevention of PTLD is possible by choosing, if possible, an EBV-negative donor. Finding an EBV-negative donor is unusual, as most of the population has been infected with EBV in the past. In most transplant recipients, the level of EBV in the blood can be followed and, if it is rising, the degree of immune suppression can be decreased as much as possible. Patients could be given monoclonal antibodies or the dose of antiviral medications could be increased.

Methotrexate-Associated Lymphoma

Methotrexate is a chemotherapy drug that also suppresses the immune system. It is often used to treat autoimmune disorders such as rheumatoid arthritis. In addition to the immunosuppression, this drug encourages EBV proliferation and, therefore, increases one's risk of lymphoma. If lymphoma does develop, methotrexate will generally need to be stopped. Chemotherapy and monoclonal antibodies may also be necessary after withdrawing from that drug.

30. What are T-cell lymphomas?

T-cell lymphomas are less common than B-cell lymphomas. They account for about 12% of all lymphomas. There are many different types of T-cell lymphoma listed in the updated WHO classification (see Table 3 on page 34).

31. What is peripheral T-cell lymphoma (NOS)?

Peripheral T-cell lymphoma (NOS) is the most common type of T-cell lymphoma. In addition to lymph node involvement, it is not unusual to have involvement of the liver, spleen, and bone marrow. Rashes due to lymphoma involvement also occur. This type of lymphoma tends to be more aggressive than the equivalent B-cell lymphoma (DLBCL-NOS). This may be due to a higher frequency of patients presenting with higher risk features, including stage IV disease, B symptoms, and a higher serum LDH. This type of lymphoma is most common in patients in their 60s.

32. What is angioimmunoblastic T-cell lymphoma?

Angioimmunoblastic T-cell lymphoma is another type of aggressive T-cell lymphoma. It is a rare disorder, but one of the more common types of T-cell lymphoma. It usually affects older males. Typically, many lymph nodes will be enlarged, and patients may have B symptoms that include fevers, night sweats, and weight loss. It is also not uncommon for this to be associated with a rash and with autoimmune manifestations. Rheumatologic abnormalities may occur, including joint pain and swelling (arthritis). Frequently, there will be a high level of immunoglobulins detected in the blood (hypergamma-globulinemia). EBV is felt to be involved in many of these cases.

33. What is anaplastic large cell lymphoma (ALK-positive and ALK-negative)?

Anaplastic large cell lymphoma can be either ALK-positive or ALK-negative. This is a rare type of lymphoma, accounting for 2–3% of all lymphomas and about 8–10% of all T-cell lymphomas. It usually presents with lymph node enlargement. The protein CD30 is found on the surface of the cells. This protein is also normally found in Hodgkin lymphoma. Apart from lymph nodes, other sites can also be affected, and this is more likely to occur in the more aggressive ALK-negative type. The ALK protein can be identified in the cytoplasm and on the nuclei in ALK-positive cases. It results from a chromosomal translocation and, when present, may be associated with a less aggressive clinical course. ALK-positive patients usually respond better to treatment. ALK is usually positive in younger patients, including children, and overall, 50–80% of patients with anaplastic large cell lymphoma are ALK-positive.

ALK is usually positive in younger patients, including children, and overall, 50–80% of patients with anaplastic large cell lymphoma are ALK-positive.

34. What is adult T-cell lymphoma/leukemia?

Adult T-cell lymphoma/leukemia is caused by HTLV-1. This virus commonly affects people living in the Caribbean or southwestern Japan, and also the southeastern US. Only 2–3% of people infected with this virus will develop adult T-cell lymphoma/leukemia, and then, only usually after being infected for between 10 and 40 years. The virus can also cause a neurologic disorder called tropical spastic paraparesis. This lymphoma/leukemia can present in either an acute or chronic form, and there are 4 different types. When it is acute, symptoms may be caused by a high calcium level, which can result in **dehydration** and confusion. Bone pain due to bone involvement can occur. Lymph node enlargement, liver and spleen involvement, and abnormally circulating lymphoma cells are common.

Dehydration

Low fluids in the body, which can cause dizziness, fatigue, fainting, and other minor symptoms. If not corrected, dehydration can cause more serious problems.

The chronic form is much less aggressive and is associated with lesser degrees of lymph node involvement and, often, a rash.

35. What are the different types of T/NK cell lymphoma, including extranodal NK/T-cell lymphoma, nasal type?

The WHO classification continues to try to make sense of the greater understanding of leukemias and lymphomas derived from T cells and NK cells. The latest version of this classification is seen in Table 3 on page 34.

T-cell large granular lymphocytic leukemia and chronic lymphoproliferative disorders of NK cells are slow growing and often may not require any specific therapy. The NK cells are a type of lymphocyte referred to as the large granular lymphocyte. Some T cells are also large granular lymphocytes. Both NK cell- and T cell-derived proliferations of large granular lymphocytes are very similar in their behavior. Most people with this disorder will have T-cell–derived leukemia cells, with the remaining 15% being of NK-cell origin. Patients will often be found to have a low blood count, with the neutrophil count being the most commonly affected. This is often associated with recurrent bacterial infections. An enlarged spleen is often present, and the liver may also be enlarged. This disorder may be associated with the development of rheumatoid arthritis or other autoimmune disorders. The bone marrow is usually also involved.

Extranodal NK/T-cell lymphoma is an aggressive type of lymphoma that originates mainly from NK cells rather than from T cells (see **Table 8**). As its name suggests, it most frequently affects the nasal cavity and sinuses. It often causes blockage of the nose, nasal discharge, or nose bleeding, and can also affect the roof of the mouth (palate) and other areas throughout the gut, skin, testes, and airway. Extranodal NK/T-cell lymphoma can also involve the orbit, causing swelling around the eye, and is associated with EBV. It is much more common in parts of Asia and, to a lesser extent, South and Central America, but rare cases also occur in the US and Europe. The nasal type is often localized to that area when first diagnosed.

36. What is enteropathy-associated T-cell lymphoma?

Enteropathy-associated T-cell lymphoma is a lymphoma that affects the small bowel. It is a rare but aggressive disorder that most commonly affects adults with celiac disease, also called gluten-sensitive enteropathy. It sometimes is diagnosed before celiac disease. Patients may present with abdominal pain, bleeding from the bowel, or a bowel obstruction.

37. What is hepatosplenic T-cell lymphoma?

Hepatosplenic T-cell lymphoma is another rare but often very aggressive type of lymphoma. Affected individuals typically present with an enlarged liver and spleen, lymphoma involving the bone marrow, and low blood counts. Lymph nodes are usually not enlarged. The lymphocytes of most patients with other types

Table 8 Leukemias and Lymphomas derived from T cells and NK (Natural Killer) cells

Leukemic or disseminated

T-cell prolymphocytic leukemia

T-cell large granular lymphocytic leukemia

Chronic lymphoproliferative disorders of NK cells*

Aggressive NK cell leukemia

Systemic Epstein-Barr virus (EBV)–positive T-cell lymphoproliferative disorders of childhood

Adult T-cell lymphoma/leukemia (HTLV-1-positive)

Extranodal

Extranodal NK/T-cell lymphoma, nasal type

Enteropathy-associated T-cell lymphoma

Hepatosplenic T-cell lymphoma

Extranodal—cutaneous

Mycosis fungoides

Sezary syndrome

Primary cutaneous CD30+ lymphoproliferative disorders

    Primary cutaneous anaplastic large cell lymphoma

    Lymphomatoid papulosis

Subcutaneous panniculitis-like T-cell lymphoma

Primary cutaneous gamma/delta T-cell lymphoma*

Primary cutaneous aggressive epidermotropic CD8+ cytotoxic T-cell lymphoma*

Primary cutaneous small/medium CD4+ T-cell lymphoma*

Nodal

Angioimmunoblastic T-cell lymphoma

Anaplastic large cell lymphoma, ALK-positive

Anaplastic large cell lymphoma, ALK-negative*

Peripheral T-cell lymphoma, not otherwise specified

* designates provisional entities

Reproduced from: The 2008 WHO classification of lymphomas: implications for clinical practice and translational research Elaine S. Jaffe Hematopathology Section, Laboratory of Pathology, Center for Cancer Research, National Cancer Institute, National Institutes of Health, Bethesda, MD ASH Education Book January 1, 2009 vol. 2009 no. 1 523-531

DIAGNOSIS AND CLASSIFICATION OF LYMPHOMA

of T-cell lymphoma will have the alpha/beta receptor identified on the surface of the abnormal lymphocytes. The abnormal lymphocytes in hepatosplenic T-cell lymphoma have the gamma/delta receptor on their surface. This can be detected by flow cytometry, the test that examines which proteins are present on the surface of cells. This lymphoma can be very difficult to treat and is often refractory to chemotherapy.

38. What lymphomas affect the skin?

Many lymphomas can affect the skin. The most common types are **mycosis fungoides** and CD30+ anaplastic large cell lymphoma. Additional lymphomas can involve the skin, as shown in Table 8 of the WHO/EORTC classification. **Subcutaneous** panniculitis-like T-cell lymphoma affects the fatty area below the actual skin, but it usually results in skin discoloration or nodules. If only skin is affected, it is a primary cutaneous lymphoma. Secondary cutaneous lymphoma implies spread from other sites, such as lymph nodes. Although most lymphomas have the potential to involve skin, this is uncommon, and lymphoma involving the skin is usually primary. Most skin lymphomas are composed of T cells, but B-cell lymphomas also occur.

The skin can be affected in a number of ways, such as a small area of redness or skin thickening in one place such as on the forehead or scalp, or many small affected areas may occur in one region, eventually merging into one larger area. Often these areas are flat or only slightly raised, but sometimes, actual nodules can appear. In some cases, the area can become very extensive. Patients often notice a skin abnormality that is changing and will see a dermatologist who may remove the lesion and send

Mycosis fungoides

A type of lymphoma that mainly involves the skin.

Subcutaneous

Underneath the skin.

Many lymphomas can affect the skin. The most common types are mycosis fungoides and CD30+ anaplastic large cell lymphoma.

it to the laboratory for a pathologist's review. If a diagnosis of lymphoma is made, patients should be evaluated for any other evidence of lymphoma. Further tests may include a bone marrow examination and CT scans.

39. What is mycosis fungoides?

Mycosis fungoides is a T-cell lymphoma that primarily affects the skin but occasionally, can spread to the lymph nodes and bone marrow. It is more common in older individuals and has a higher incidence in the African-American population. It is much less common in the Asian and Hispanic populations. It causes an itchy rash that can be very severe and bothersome. It tends to go through various stages with either flat patches of skin involvement, raised areas called plaques, development of tumors, or generalized skin redness (erythroderma) associated with skin breakdown and development of painful fissures. Patients can present with any of these stages or progress from one stage to the next. Features from different stages may be present at the same time. Patients with limited patch or plaque involvement sometimes never progress. Such individuals may live a normal life span. The presence of skin tumors, generalized erythroderma, lymphoma involving lymph nodes, or internal organs or circulating lymphoma cells (Sezary syndrome) carries a worse prognosis. The areas of skin most likely to be affected are those that typically do not receive much sun exposure: the trunk, buttocks, thighs, or upper arms. When tumors develop, the overlying skin can break down, developing ulcers. Infections resulting from skin breakdown are common in advanced stages. The skin involvement can be very extensive and can also affect the palms and soles, resulting in difficulty walking. Many patients may previously have been diagnosed with dermatitis or eczema that did not respond to treatment. Even a skin biopsy may not provide a definite diagnosis initially.

In more advanced cases, lymph nodes can be affected. Lymph node enlargement may also be a reaction to infection or inflammation rather than a result of lymphoma involvement.

40. What is Sezary syndrome?

Sezary syndrome is very similar to mycosis fungoides, but involves lymphoma cells circulating in the blood. Under the microscope, the nucleus of the cells has a similar shape to a brain, and their appearance has been termed cerebriform. Sezary syndrome may develop from preexisting mycosis fungoides or may occur without any history of mycosis fungoides.

41. What is primary cutaneous CD30+ anaplastic large cell lymphoma?

Primary cutaneous CD30+ anaplastic large cell lymphoma is uncommon. It primarily involves the skin but in some cases can spread to involve lymph nodes or organs. The skin lesions present as nodules, usually on the legs, and can be single or develop in crops. The lesions can resolve spontaneously, recurring periodically. Lesions may bleed or become infected. The diagnosis of this lymphoma is made by skin biopsy. The cells have a protein called CD30 on their surface. Under the microscope, the cells can appear identical to the appearance of another disorder called lymphomatoid papulosis, which is considered to be benign but carries a risk of transforming into lymphoma.

A number of treatment options are available, including topical steroids; topical protopic (tacrolimus), which is an immunosuppressive medication; **phototherapy**; topical retinoids; chemotherapy skin treatments; **interferon therapy**; and radiation therapy. Newer medications, including bexarotene (Targretin®), Vorinostat (Zolinza®), and denileukin diftitox (Ontak®), are also effective. Trials are also being conducted using a monoclonal antibody directed against CD30 (brentuximab vedotin).

Some lymphomas involving the skin are indolent and may not require any treatment; however, others are more aggressive, sometimes requiring an intravenous chemotherapy regimen such as **cyclophosphamide, doxorubicin, vincristine, and prednisone** (often referred to by the acronym CHOP).

42. What are the different types of Hodgkin lymphoma?

A number of subtypes of Hodgkin lymphoma exist (see Table 1 on page 19), and the pathologist distinguishes their appearance under a microscope. The two main categories are NLPHL and classical Hodgkin lymphoma. There are four different subtypes of classical Hodgkin lymphoma: **nodular sclerosis Hodgkin lymphoma, mixed cellularity Hodgkin lymphoma, lymphocyte-rich Hodgkin lymphoma**, and **lymphocyte-depleted Hodgkin lymphoma**. Unlike non-Hodgkin lymphomas, the malignant or cancerous cell may actually be difficult to find, as very few may be present and are greatly outnumbered by normal cells. The normal cells seen are those usually found in conditions of infection or inflammation. The number and types of the normal

DIAGNOSIS AND CLASSIFICATION OF LYMPHOMA

Phototherapy
A type of therapy using ultraviolet light.

Interferon therapy
A type of immune therapy.

Cyclophosphamide, doxorubicin, vincristine, and prednisone
Four drugs that are commonly used together to treat lymphoma.

Nodular sclerosis Hodgkin lymphoma
The most common type of Hodgkin lymphoma.

Mixed cellularity Hodgkin lymphoma
One of the types of Hodgkin lymphoma.

Lymphocyte-rich Hodgkin lymphoma
A type of Hodgkin lymphoma.

Lymphocyte-depleted Hodgkin lymphoma
A type of Hodgkin lymphoma.

cells, the surface protein expression on those cells, and the amount of scar tissue present in the lymph node will determine what type of Hodgkin lymphoma is present.

Nodular Lymphocyte–Predominant Hodgkin Lymphoma (NLPHL)

NLPHL differs from classical Hodgkin lymphoma and is derived from a B-cell and often behaves like an indolent B-cell lymphoma. It is usually fairly localized at diagnosis and more commonly affect males. Options for management include watchful waiting, radiotherapy, anti-CD20 directed monoclonal antibodies, or chemotherapy. These treatments can be used alone or in combination. As can happen with other types of indolent B-cell lymphomas, this type of Hodgkin lymphoma carries the risk of transformation to a higher-grade lymphoma, often to a T-cell/histiocyte-rich B-cell lymphoma.

Classical Hodgkin Lymphoma

Nodular sclerosis Hodgkin lymphoma is the most common type, accounting for 75% of cases. It occurs more commonly in females and frequently involves the mediastinal lymph nodes, which are situated in the center of the chest between the lungs. Commonly, neck lymph nodes will also be enlarged. When the biopsy specimen is examined under the microscope, thick bands of scar tissue (**fibrosis**) are seen surrounding the lymphocytes and inflammatory cells. Most patients have stage II disease at diagnosis, meaning at least two lymph node areas are involved on the same side of the diaphragm.

Mixed cellularity Hodgkin lymphoma is another subtype that accounts for 25–30% of cases. It is more common in men, can be quite aggressive at the time

The number and types of the normal cells, the surface protein expression on those cells, and the amount of scar tissue present in the lymph node will determine what type of Hodgkin lymphoma is present.

Fibrosis

The replacement of normal tissue with scar tissue.

of diagnosis, and is frequently associated with bone marrow involvement; B symptoms are not uncommon.

Lymphocyte-rich Hodgkin lymphoma is also more common in men than in women and accounts for 5% of cases. This type of lymphoma may have the **CD20** protein on its surface. As a result, monoclonal antibodies may have a role in treatment under some circumstances. This type of lymphoma can behave in an indolent fashion, similar to the indolent non-Hodgkin lymphomas.

CD20

A protein on the surface of B-lymphocytes and most B-cell lymphomas.

The final and least common subtype is lymphocyte-depleted Hodgkin lymphoma, which generally behaves as a more aggressive type of lymphoma. It only accounts for about 1% of cases.

PART THREE

Staging and Treatment of Lymphoma

What happens after I'm told that
I have lymphoma?

Should I get a second opinion?

Apart from the biopsy, what other
information is needed?

More . . .

43. What happens after I'm told that I have lymphoma?

Hearing that you have lymphoma, as with any form of serious illness or cancer, can be a frightening and overwhelming experience. For many people, it is the first serious illness that they have faced, and many different emotions may arise. Patients often experience the various stages that are commonly associated with the grieving process, namely denial, anger, bargaining, **depression**, and finally, acceptance. The duration and intensity of the different stages vary among individuals.

The surgeon who performed the biopsy is the first person to receive the results, which will be discussed with you at your first follow-up visit; however, many surgeons may not feel comfortable addressing the multitude of questions that are foremost in your mind. An appointment will be arranged with a lymphoma specialist, who can provide you with some answers. Whenever possible, this appointment should take place sooner rather than later so that your questions can be answered to help minimize your anxiety and fears.

A lymphoma specialist is a physician who is trained in **hematology** or **oncology**—and frequently both of these specialties. A hematologist has received specialty training in the management of blood disorders, including cancers related to the blood and lymphatic systems, such as lymphoma, leukemia, and multiple myeloma. An oncologist is a specialist who is trained in the management of all cancers in general. Most hematology and oncology training programs in the US are combined, and, as a result, most lymphoma patients receive treatment from a physician trained in both of these specialties. In communities with a university teaching hospital,

Depression

A disorder characterized by excessive sadness and feelings of hopelessness.

Hematology

The study of diseases of the blood, including blood cancers.

Oncology

The field of medicine that studies cancer.

there are often groups of physicians who specialize in mainly lymphoma or mainly leukemia.

The first step in coming to terms with the diagnosis is arming yourself with information and deciding on a plan of management. Therefore, hopefully, your appointment with the lymphoma specialist can be expedited. For the first appointment, it is a good idea to bring your spouse, a close relative, or a friend to provide much-needed emotional support, to remember to ask helpful questions, and to help in remembering the details. You may also find it helpful to record the meeting, as a lot of information can be discussed at that first appointment. Before your appointment, your primary care doctor or surgeon will generally send or fax your medical records, including the biopsy results, to the lymphoma specialist's office. This allows your lymphoma doctor to review your information before the meeting. The benefit is that more time from the appointment can be dedicated to discussion about the nature of lymphoma, what other tests are needed, and how best to treat the disease. Your specialist will wish to review the symptoms that you have been experiencing and also obtain additional information about your past medical history. Because you have likely told the same story to a number of doctors and nurses previously, this can seem very repetitive; however, to ensure that nothing gets missed, this process is very important and is usually time well spent for both you and your new physician. This allows you and your doctor to get to know each other better.

At the initial visit, you may first meet with a nurse or medical assistant who will obtain some baseline information. After filling out a form that provides details of your past medical and surgical history, family history, medications, and any drug allergies, you then will

The most important parts of the examination are the lymph nodes, liver, and spleen, but a general examination is also important in evaluating any other areas that the lymphoma may be affecting and what these effects might be, as well as to get a sense of your overall health.

meet with the lymphoma doctor, who will ask questions about your symptoms and how you are currently feeling. You will then change into a gown to be examined. Gynecologic and rectal examinations are usually not required. The most important parts of the examination are the lymph nodes, liver, and spleen, but a general examination is also important in evaluating any other areas that the lymphoma may be affecting and what these effects might be, as well as to get a sense of your overall health.

This information is vital for deciding on the appropriate treatment. You may or may not prefer having your friend or relative remain in the room during the appointment or examination.

After the examination, your doctor will discuss lymphoma in general and your lymphoma in particular. Other required tests, including blood tests, scans, and usually a bone marrow examination, will give a complete picture of the extent of the lymphoma. A full discussion of the stage of the lymphoma and a treatment plan may need to wait for the next visit after the tests are completed. At that time, enough information will be available to allow for a more detailed discussion of your particular lymphoma. If possible, it is better not to discuss too much information at that first visit, especially if you are hearing the diagnosis for the first time. At the time of the next visit, your thinking may be much clearer, and you may be able to absorb a lot more information. Your doctor may also be able to provide you with some reading material relating to lymphoma or useful Web sites to visit for more information.

44. Should I get a second opinion?

A second opinion is a good idea if there is any doubt regarding the correct diagnosis, if you have any concerns about the proposed treatment, or if you do not feel comfortable about any aspects of the information or care plan you received from your first lymphoma doctor. Most insurance companies will cover a second opinion. It is a good idea to check with your insurance carrier to see if any restrictions apply. You do not want to be surprised by any out-of-pocket expenses.

If there is doubt regarding the diagnosis, you may request that another pathologist review the slides. In most cases, however, as long as adequate material has been obtained for review by the pathologist, the diagnosis is not likely to be in doubt, and often, more than one of the pathologists within the department will have already examined the slides. It can be comforting, however, to receive confirmation of the diagnosis and treatment options from another lymphoma specialist. Sometimes seeking a second opinion may result in transferring your care to the new doctor, depending on your preference and the options that your insurance company will allow. In any event, your first lymphoma doctor should be comfortable in having you seek a second opinion if you wish. Usually, his or her office will give you a copy of all relevant material, including clinic notes and pathology reports from the lymph node and bone marrow biopsies and any radiology studies, such as CT and PET scans. The doctor who provides the second opinion will require these reports and will probably also need to have the actual biopsy slides and X-rays/scans evaluated at the hospital to ensure that the advice given is based on accurate information.

It is important to recognize that there are many acceptable options and often more than one correct option for dealing with a diagnosis of lymphoma. You may, therefore, receive different recommendations from different physicians, with none of them being wrong. Some patients may then seek a third opinion, getting yet another set of recommendations. If you feel comfortable with your first physician and all of your questions have been answered satisfactorily, second opinions may really be unnecessary and may lead to delays in proceeding with treatment as you attempt to sort all of the different options.

45. Apart from the biopsy, what other information is needed?

As mentioned previously, after the first time you see your lymphoma specialist, additional tests will need to be performed. These tests are needed to determine the answers to several questions. First, what is the stage of your lymphoma? This relates to which body parts are affected. A good diagnostic quality contrast-enhanced CT scan or a PET/CT scan is usually obtained to examine the lymph nodes in the chest, abdomen, and pelvis. A bone marrow biopsy is performed to evaluate the bone marrow for the presence of lymphoma.

Other tests performed much less frequently include an MRI, a lymphangiogram and a gallium scan. These tests are discussed in Question 15 on page 37 and can provide important information in some cases. Other tests are performed to provide information on how your particular lymphoma is likely to behave over time—in other words, to determine the likely prognosis. Question 19 on page 49 describes how, in general, indolent lymphomas can be quite slow growing and can be managed with intermittent treatment over fairly long periods of time; however, while this is true in the average patient with indolent lymphoma, there may be certain features specific to you that give a better idea of whether your lymphoma will be more or less aggressive. The features that are useful for determining the prognosis have been pooled together into prognostic indices. For indolent lymphoma, the **Follicular Lymphoma International Prognostic Index (FLIPI)** (see Question 47 on page 103) is used. For aggressive lymphomas, the **International Prognostic Index (IPI)** is used (see Question 46 on page 100). For mantle cell lymphoma, the Mantle Cell Lymphoma Prognostic Index (MIPI), devised by a German group, is more useful than either the IPI or FLIPI for providing prognostic information on this type of lymphoma. More studies are needed before the MIPI is used to decide on treatment. All of this information can be obtained from the patient's general physical health status, scans, blood tests, and bone marrow examination.

In certain situations, it may be important that blood tests for hepatitis B, hepatitis C, and HIV are performed. Other information needed will depend on your general health apart from the lymphoma. This information is important in determining your ability to tolerate the various treatment options. For example, your doctor may need to evaluate how well your heart is functioning, as some chemotherapy drugs used to treat lymphoma can affect heart function. If there is any concern about the ability of your heart to tolerate that treatment, an alternative chemotherapy drug may be chosen. Similarly, special breathing tests, called **pulmonary function tests**, may be required, as some drugs can cause lung damage. The risk of lung damage may

Follicular Lymphoma International Prognostic Index (FLIPI)

A modified form of the IPI for determining the prognosis of patients with follicular lymphomas.

International Prognostic Index (IPI)

A system to determine the prognosis of patients with lymphoma.

Pulmonary function tests

A set of tests performed to evaluate the ability of the lungs to function properly.

be higher if your lung function is not optimal before beginning chemotherapy.

All of this information is generally obtained before starting treatment for the lymphoma. After the test results are available, your doctor will schedule another appointment to discuss the results and treatment plan with you.

Many types of chemotherapy have a temporary or permanent effect on fertility. It is reasonable for younger patients, both males and females, to seek reproductive counseling when time allows for this.

46. What is the IPI?

The IPI is a method that is used to estimate a statistical chance of how well you will do with treatment. It was first introduced for the aggressive lymphomas but appears to be also useful for many other types of non-Hodgkin lymphomas. First introduced in 1993, it has gained wide acceptance but is limited in terms of its ability to be useful in planning treatment of lymphoma. In large studies from the US, Canada, and Europe, a number of features associated with many patients diagnosed with lymphoma were documented and then correlated with the results of treatment. After the analysis was completed, it was seen that five specific features were important, independent of each other, and when combined, allowed separation of patients into better and poorer prognosis groups. Another group with an intermediate prognosis was also identified. It is important to understand that all of the elements of the various prognostic scoring systems are obtained prior to any therapy being started. These systems were all therefore designed to give "snapshot" probabilities of the outcome with treatment before any actual treatment began.

The following features that are helpful for determining prognosis were combined into this IPI: (1) age, (2) stage, (3) serum **lactate dehydrogenase (LDH)**, (4) **performance status**, and (5) extranodal involvement. These features require further explanation. Older patients in general fare worse than younger ones; therefore, being older than 60 receives one point in the index. Second, patients with stage I or stage II disease generally do better than patients with stage III or stage IV disease; therefore, stage III or stage IV disease receives another point. The third feature is the level of LDH in the bloodstream. LDH is present in red blood cells, liver, bone, and many other tissues. It is frequently increased in patients with lymphoma and reflects the body's "burden" of lymphoma and the rate at which it is growing. A level above normal is an additional risk factor and receives another point. Another point is given if the lymphoma involves sites other than the lymph nodes (so-called extranodal sites) including the bone marrow, gut, liver, lung, and CNS (including the brain, spinal cord, and/or spinal fluid). A final feature in the IPI is the performance status, which is a measure of how well one is able to carry out one's everyday activities. The Eastern Cooperative Oncology Group scale is shown in **Table 9**. Other scoring systems, such as the **Karnofsky Performance Status scale**, are also used to evaluate the level of functioning. Another point is given for patients with a score of 2 to 4.

Thus, because there are five features in the IPI, any patient can have a score of 0 to 5, but most patients have a score of between 0 and 3. The score allows your doctor to estimate your likely response to treatment. The likelihood of success of therapy is greatest with a lower score. Patients with higher scores may also do very well, as these likelihoods are statistical and may not apply to individual

STAGING AND TREATMENT OF LYMPHOMA

Lactate dehydrogenase (LDH)

An enzyme measured using a simple blood test.

Performance status

The level of ability with which patients can perform their routine daily activities.

Karnofsky Performance Status scale

A system to evaluate how patients do when performing normal daily activities.

Table 9 Eastern Cooperative Oncology Group Performance Status Scale

0	No symptoms; fully active; able to carry out all normal activities.
1	Symptoms present but able to carry out normal activities; some difficulty with more strenuous activities.
2	Able to carry out normal self-care activities but limited in ability to work; up and about more than 50% of the time.
3	Capable of only limited self-care; confined to bed or chair more than 50% of waking hours.
4	Completely disabled; needing full-time assistance with normal self-care activities.

Modified from: Oken, M.M., Creech, R.H., Tormey, D.C., Horton, J., Davis, T.E., McFadden, E.T., Carbone, P.P.: Toxicity And Response Criteria Of The Eastern Cooperative Oncology Group. *Am J Clin Oncol* 5:649–655, 1982. Eastern Cooperative Oncology Group, Robert Comis M.D., Group Chair.

patients. If you are younger than age 60, the presence of lymphoma in sites other than the lymph nodes doesn't result in a worse prognosis. As a result, a modification to the IPI was made, resulting in the age-adjusted IPI. This relies on only three factors to determine the prognosis: stage, LDH, and performance status.

An example of how this information is important relates to decisions regarding treatment. If you have a higher score on the IPI, you may wish to consider other treatments that may be available only through participation in a clinical trial. The IPI is also useful to ensure that patients being treated in a clinical trial where two treatments are being compared have similar characteristics. This ensures that any difference found between the two treatments is related to the treatment and not to differences in the patients who were treated in each group. It is important to realize that the IPI was developed for aggressive lymphomas, such as DLBLC-NOS.

The IPI was designed prior to the availability of monoclonal antibodies. This means that the outcomes were measured using patients who had not received monoclonal antibodies as part of their therapy. It has since been shown that the IPI still predicts outcomes for patients receiving monoclonal antibody–based therapy.

Another feature that is not included in the IPI is gene expression. This is measured by a test called gene expression profiling (GEP), a test that is becoming more widely available. It can identify a biological factor that separates patients into two groups based on the cell of origin of the lymphoma. One group has germinal centre B-cell–like lymphoma cells (GCB) and the other group has activated B-cell–like lymphoma cells (ABC). GCB lymphomas have a better prognosis than ABC lymphomas. GEP information is not generally used presently for initial therapy decisions, but as more information becomes available from clinical trials of existing and new therapies this information may help tailor treatment decisions in the future.

47. What are the Follicular Lymphoma International Prognostic Indices (FLIPI and FLIPI-2)?

The prognostic indices specific to follicular lymphomas, FLIPI and FLIPI-2, are similar to the IPI and are used to estimate prognosis for indolent lymphomas. Like the IPI, the FLIPI has gained widespread acceptance. The IPI was somewhat helpful when deciding on prognoses for indolent lymphoma patients but did not discriminate indolent lymphoma groups with differing outcomes as well as the FLIPI. They are not particularly helpful for deciding whether someone needs to commence therapy or for deciding on a specific type of therapy, and, similar to the IPI, FLIPI is more useful for interpreting the results of large clinical studies. They can, however, be helpful to patients in considering their treatment options and outlook, as mentioned in the clinical trial example previously.

The FLIPI was introduced in 2004. The same group devised a second prognostic index, the FLIPI-2, after monoclonal antibodies were introduced for treatment of lymphoma. This was introduced in 2009. As most patients now receive monoclonal antibodies, the FLIPI-2 index appears to be better and is intended for patients with larger tumor burdens.

Both indices are used and details follow. As with the IPI, the FLIPI includes five prognostic or predictive criteria. However, the FLIPI adapts these criteria to reflect the specific features known to affect the prognosis in follicular lymphoma. These criteria include: (1) more than four nodal areas, (2) elevated serum LDH levels, (3) age older than 60 years, (4) stage III or IV, and (5) anemia defined as a hemoglobin less than 12 g/dL. Scoring is performed in the same manner as with the IPI, with a score of 0–1 being considered low risk, and a score of 3–5 being considered higher risk.

The FLIPI and FLIPI-2 overlap. The FLIPI-2 contains other things that affect the prognosis. The criteria are: (1) any lymph node greater than 6 cm, (2) an elevated β-2 microglobulin (measured by a blood test), (3) being over the age of 60 years, (4) having bone marrow involvement, (5) anemia defined as a hemoglobin less than 12 g/dL.

One final note about these scores and prognostic indicators: you must always remember that they are an estimate of how you might respond given your circumstances, and they should be considered in determining how to manage

One final note about these scores and prognostic indicators: you must always remember that they are an estimate of how you might respond given your circumstances, and they should be considered in determining how to manage your particular lymphoma and your long-term prognosis, but cannot be used to decide on any particular treatment plan.

your particular lymphoma and your long-term prognosis, but cannot be used to decide on any particular treatment plan. They do not in any way predict the future perfectly for any individual patient, nor are they a statistic that dooms you to certain death or certain recovery. Patients with a poor prognosis according to these indicators often do survive lymphoma. It is important that you do not give up simply because you're facing a more daunting life-threatening challenge. Some of the more aggressive lymphomas are also some of the most curable types of cancer. Survival depends a great deal on determination to take your treatment seriously and to work hard to maintain and improve your health status. On the other hand, patients with a good prognosis could misinterpret this estimate as a guarantee of survival; if they do not pay close attention to their treatment regimen and overall health, they could find themselves facing mortal illness. Thus, it is important to understand that these indicators are a guideline for treatment, not a crystal ball, and that you should not allow them to alter your determination to beat your lymphoma (**Tables 10** and **11**).

Table 10 IPI Prognostic Factors

- Age older than 60 years
- Eastern Cooperative Oncology Group performance score of 2 or more
- Elevated lactate dehydrogenase
- More than one site of extranodal involvement
- Stage III or stage IV lymphoma

Table 11 IPI Risk Categories

Risk category	IPI risk factors
Low	0 or 1
Low–intermediate	2
High–intermediate	3
High	4 or 5

48. Is there a prognostic index for Hodgkin lymphoma?

Hodgkin lymphoma is quite different from non-Hodgkin lymphoma, and, as a result, different features are considered in its prognostic indices. There are two common prognostic systems used in Hodgkin lymphoma. The first is used for patients with limited stage (stage I or II) disease. Patients with early stage favorable disease have *none* of the following: B symptoms, a large mass (defined various ways), extranodal sites of disease, sedimentation rate greater than or equal to 50 millimeters per hour, or more than two sites of disease defined by regional lymph node groups. Differences between favorable and unfavorable disease can in some instances alter the treatment plan. An additional prognostic model using primarily patients with advanced stage disease was published in the *New England Journal of Medicine* in 1998. Factors shown to be important for a less favorable outcome in this index were being male, having stage IV disease, having a low level of **albumin** (a protein that a simple blood test measures), having anemia with a hemoglobin level of less than 10.5 g/dL, having a white count above 15,000, and finally, having a low level of lymphocytes in the blood. As noted in the previous question, having a higher number of features does not guarantee a worse outcome or that the likelihood of recurrence will be greater, but consideration may be given to more aggressive initial therapy to minimize this risk. Treatment may be tailored differently to take into account a higher risk of relapse, and, again, patients with higher scores may benefit from seeking treatment in a clinical trial. An increasing number of chemotherapy treatment regimens are available for the initial management of Hodgkin lymphoma. Choosing the correct regimen for the individual patient

Albumin

A special type of protein found in the bloodstream.

is important because with the high rate of cure, a regimen that is overly aggressive can result in increased side effects without an increase in the likelihood of cure.

49. Are all types of lymphoma treated the same way?

Quite simply, the answer is no. As there are many different types of lymphoma, the approach to treatment depends on many factors including whether the goal is cure or disease control. Even if the lymphoma is considered incurable, many different treatments are available that can control the lymphoma, often for very long periods of time. These treatments given intermittently can be very effective for disease control, keeping lymphoma patients feeling well, often for many years. Especially in recent years, a large number of newer treatments have become available for lymphoma patients, and the outlook continues to improve at a rapid rate.

Newer techniques are becoming available to better distinguish between types of lymphoma that appear to be similar. Two patients may have a lymphoma that appears to be similar, yet with the same treatment, they may respond quite differently. At least some of the explanation for this lies in differences in which types of proteins are being produced by the lymphoma cells. Certain proteins may cause a lymphoma to grow more rapidly or be resistant to a particular treatment. These proteins are determined by genes that can be turned on or off in lymphoma cells. Analyzing these genes can help to better determine the features of the lymphoma and, it is hoped, to choose better treatments on the basis of this information. Gene chip technology is the method used to evaluate which genes, and therefore which proteins, are turned on in lymphoma cells. It is currently a research technique, but many studies are clearly demonstrating its importance in the management of lymphoma. It will be very important in the near future for helping to choose the correct treatment for different patients who appear to have the same type of lymphoma.

50. What types of treatment are available for lymphoma?

The options available for the management of lymphoma include observation, monoclonal antibody therapy, radioimmunotherapy, newer specific inhibitors of molecular activity inside lymphoma cells (e.g., proteasome inhibitors such as bortezomib or Bruton's tyrosine kinase inhibitors such as ibrutinib), and chemotherapy with a number of different classes of drugs that have differing mechanisms of action and can be given either orally or by the intravenous route. External beam radiation can also be very useful in certain situations. Combinations of these different options are often administered together.

Chemotherapy refers to the use of certain classes of drugs, usually given by mouth or in a vein (intravenously). After administration, the chemotherapy enters the bloodstream and travels to every part of the body. It can be given as either one drug alone (single-agent chemotherapy) or combined with other chemotherapy drugs (combination chemotherapy). A perfect chemotherapy drug would damage only cancer cells, but most drugs in use today can also damage normal cells, resulting in side effects. Certain chemotherapy drugs can also be given in very high doses, producing a greater effect against the lymphoma, but the most important side effect of this would be an increased degree of destruction of the bone marrow. Giving high-dose chemotherapy along with the infusion of bone marrow stem cells is the basis for bone marrow or stem cell transplantation (discussed in Question 82 on page 173). Radiation, another type of treatment, is usually given to specific areas of the body affected by lymphoma in order to control disease at that location. Sometimes it is administered to areas more prominently affected by the lymphoma after the administration of chemotherapy that was given to control more generalized disease. In this situation, it is used in an attempt to prevent the lymphoma from coming back at a particular site after treatment with chemotherapy.

51. How is indolent lymphoma treated?

After diagnosis and staging, the next step is to make decisions about treatment. As strange as it may seem, one commonly used option is something called "watch and wait." Other options include receiving a monoclonal antibody alone or combined with chemotherapy. The chemotherapy can be given as pills or as intravenous chemotherapy, of which there is a growing list of options. Other options include radiotherapy and transplant options. All of these options may be acceptable depending on the specific features of an individual patient's lymphoma, what treatment has previously been administered, and also the patient's personal preferences. You can discuss the merits of each of these approaches with your lymphoma doctor.

The watch-and-wait concept has been around for many years and arose from observations that the indolent lymphomas often are slow growing, frequently not associated with any symptoms, and can generally be controlled with therapy when it is necessary to prevent the lymphoma from causing problems. Earlier treatment has not yet been shown to prolong survival. Furthermore, as some treatments can have long-term harmful effects, saving their use for later when they may be more necessary helps to minimize this. Also, accepting watch and wait carries with it the understanding that the indolent lymphomas are not generally considered curable with conventional doses of chemotherapy. Additional reasons to consider the watch-and-wait approach include the possible side effects from chemotherapy and also that the chemotherapy drugs work best the first time they are used. Therefore, keeping the drugs in reserve until symptoms or problems occur or seem likely to occur may be a valid strategy. Not every patient is comfortable with this approach, and indeed, some physicians feel that this is a defeatist attitude. Certainly, if you feel uncomfortable with this approach, you should discuss your feelings with your physician or obtain a second opinion. If symptoms are present or if the lymph node enlargement is causing problems, treatment will generally be recommended. Monoclonal antibodies have been introduced long after people were managed with the watch-and-wait option. The obvious question is whether patients with indolent lymphoma should be treated with monoclonal antibodies instead of a watch-and-wait approach. The answer depends on a number of features but certain points need to be considered. Watch-and wait is not appropriate for people with bulky lymph nodes/high tumor burden or symptoms associated with the lymphoma. Indolent lymphoma is generally considered incurable with standard doses of chemotherapy/ monoclonal antibody therapy and the disease tends to be controllable when treatment is finally administered. Using the watch-and-wait approach, there can be quite a long period, often measured in years, before treatment is needed. A small proportion of patients may never require therapy for an indolent lymphoma. Studies have indicated no survival benefit between the watch-and-wait approach versus receiving monoclonal antibodies at the time of diagnosis. In patients receiving monoclonal antibodies at the time of diagnosis, there will be a longer time before patients notice lymphoma progression and/or will need to receive further treatment. However, if you do not have bulky disease or symptoms, delaying this benefit will do no harm. This benefit will most likely occur when the treatment is actually given. This allows you to avoid any adverse events from the treatment and continue living as normal, without treatment.

A reason to avoid the watch-and-wait approach is if it is causing undue anxiety. Most people, after they have had a good conversation with their physician, will understand the reasons behind the watch-and-wait approach and feel comfortable with it.

When the watch-and-wait approach is chosen, you should be seen on a regular basis by your lymphoma specialist. You should be alert for any symptoms that could indicate progression of lymphoma. Blood counts should be checked regularly, because any fall in the blood counts could signal disease progression or occasionally immunologic complications of the lymphoma. Most patients, however, need some form of treatment after a few months to 3 years.

In our opinion, watch and wait will continue to be a very sensible option until it can be scientifically shown that patients treated sooner actually survive longer than those who receive no immediate treatment at the time of their diagnosis.

If the decision is made to proceed with treatment, many options are available (shown in **Table 12**).

Traditionally, chemotherapy was the first treatment that most patients with indolent lymphoma received. More recently, monoclonal antibodies alone or given along with chemotherapy have become a common first-line therapy. The challenge is to select the right agent or combination of agents best suited to the patient's circumstances (specific chemotherapy drugs are discussed in Question 60 on page 135). As noted previously, the approach to treating indolent lymphoma differs among physicians. A common and widely accepted initial therapy is a monoclonal antibody (rituximab) combined with cyclophosphamide, vincristine, and prednisone (R-CVP). Another option is a monoclonal antibody combined with cyclophosphamide, vincristine and prednisone in addition to doxorubicin. The most common monoclonal antibody used is rituximab and this regimen is termed the R-CHOP regimen. The choice between these regimens is often based only on physician preference, with some preferring to save the doxorubicin, an anthracycline chemotherapy agent, for a future treatment. The rationale for this staged approach is to use less chemotherapy early, when the lymphoma

Table 12 Options Available for the Treatment of Indolent Lymphoma

Watch and wait

Chemotherapy pills

Intravenous chemotherapy in combination

Localized radiation (rarely)

Monoclonal antibody therapy

Radioimmunotherapy

Autologous stem cell transplant

Allogeneic stem cell transplant

is the most responsive to chemotherapy. Over time, the lymphoma is likely to be more resistant to chemotherapy, and stronger regimens will be needed. Giving stronger chemotherapy earlier has not been shown to prolong survival over milder chemotherapy and may add additional side effects that may cause more serious problems in later years or may interfere with quality of life.

On the other hand, many physicians feel that a more intensive treatment, although more likely to cause side effects, will produce a longer remission. This may allow patients to go longer before needing another type of treatment. One downside of this is that it is unlikely that, after receiving the more intensive treatments, the patients will subsequently respond to less intensive treatments. Certain patients will benefit from the less intensive treatments, often for many years, and the FLIPI or the FLIPI-2 or other measures may, in the future, allow such patients to be identified, thereby sparing them from the premature introduction of overly aggressive treatments.

Fludarabine is another useful drug if you have indolent lymphoma. It is often used in combination with other chemotherapy and/or monoclonal antibodies for the progression of the lymphoma occurring after treatment with monoclonal antibodies and CHOP. The CHOP regimen may not be recommended for some patients because of its effect on heart function; fludarabine may thus be a reasonable choice for these patients. Because fludarabine depresses the immune system, you need to be especially watchful for any signs of infection. Because of its effect on the bone marrow, it can potentially be more difficult to collect bone marrow stem cells for an autologous transplant after treatment with fludarabine. Fludarabine is often administered along with rituximab and sometimes also cyclophosphamide in a regimen called FCR, as well as with other chemotherapy agents.

Other treatments that have been developed and studied in indolent lymphoma are the radioimmunotherapy agents ^{131}I tositumomab (Bexxar) and ^{90}Y ibritumomab tiuxetan (Zevalin). These are treatments that are related to rituximab. They differ from rituximab primarily in that they have a radioactive molecule attached to the antibody (radioactive iodine or ^{131}I for Bexxar and radioactive yttrium or ^{90}Y for Zevalin). As a result, the radioactivity is carried directly to the lymphoma. It was hoped that these types of radioimmunotherapy agents would be more effective than rituximab. However clinical trials failed to show a clear consistent advantage for these agents compared to rituximab. Also with the ease of administration of rituximab compared to the comparatively more complicated administration of radioimmunotherapy agents, their use has not become so widespread as expected. The company that makes ^{131}I tositumomab decided to withdraw their agent from the market in 2014. ^{90}Y ibritumomab tiuxetan remains available and is approved for relapsed or refractory indolent or follicular B-cell lymphomas and for patients with previously untreated follicular lymphoma who achieve a response to initial chemotherapy.

The availability of monoclonal antibodies has dramatically changed the way that many types of lymphoma are treated. These agents are effective and well tolerated, and are being increasingly used as one of the first treatments administered for indolent lymphoma. Rituximab, as previously noted, can also safely be combined with many chemotherapy regimens without any significant increase in side effects, and appears to improve the results over the use of chemotherapy alone.

Another relatively new option for patients with indolent lymphoma is bendamustine. This is a drug with an interesting history. It was originally developed in East Germany in the early 1960s and was used behind the Iron Curtain for a number of malignancies including CLL, non-Hodgkin lymphoma, Hodgkin lymphoma, multiple myeloma, and breast cancer. After German unification, controlled clinical trials were performed in Europe as well as in North America that demonstrated the effectiveness of bendamustine, resulting in its approval by the Food and Drug Administration (FDA) for treatment of indolent lymphoma that has progressed after prior treatment with rituximab or a rituximab-containing therapy. Bendamustine rarely causes hair loss and is generally well tolerated, and has been a valuable addition to the options available for treatment of indolent lymphoma. Present data suggests that for indolent lymphomas the combination of bendamustine and rituimab is likely at least as effective (with fewer side effects) as CHOP plus rituximab.

Another concept in the treatment of indolent lymphomas is that of maintenance therapy. The idea behind maintenance therapy is to continue treatment with some form after the patient is in remission with the hope that it will prolong the duration of remission. Present data demonstrates that maintenance therapy with rituximab can prolong remissions in patients after initial or subsequent treatment of an indolent lymphoma. However, it has not been shown that this makes patients live longer or attain cure. It appears that patients on maintenance therapy may get infections more easily. It is also possible that the same "gains" offered by maintenance therapy could be made up for that patient in the future with their next treatment. Finally, it should be understood that there is a very remote but possible association between rituximab and a nervous system illness known as progressive multifocal leukoencephalopathy (PML). This illness is the result of reactivation of a quiescent viral infection in the brain and is observed most often in very immunosuppressed patients. The incidence of this in patients treated with rituximab is extremely low—much less than even one percent—and although the association does not prove rituximab causes PML, it is worthwhile for patients to understand this as a remote possibility when considering the use of additional rituximab such as with maintenance therapy, particularly when no clear survival advantage comes from the use of maintenance therapy. Trials also demonstrate that the use of radioimmunotherapy at the end of chemotherapy (i.e., as consolidation of the chemotherapy treatment) can produce similar gains as maintenance rituximab.

High-dose therapy refers to the administration of very intensive chemotherapy with or without radiation. Because these high doses that are designed to maximally reduce the lymphoma also destroy the patient's own bone marrow, they are generally given in conjunction with an autologous stem cell transplant (discussed in Questions 83 and 84 on pages 175 and 177). The higher treatment doses may result in a longer remission in certain patients, but, unfortunately, this strategy does not likely offer a cure for the majority of patients with indolent lymphoma.

An allogeneic transplant offers a different approach against lymphoma. This treatment option can potentially cure indolent lymphomas.

An allogeneic transplant offers a different approach against lymphoma. This treatment option can potentially cure indolent lymphomas. This treatment uses bone marrow or peripheral blood stem cells from a brother or sister or sometimes from an unrelated individual. Because there are significant risks associated with an allogeneic transplant, it is not a suitable treatment option for most patients with indolent lymphoma, and for appropriate candidates it takes a great deal of consideration and understanding on the part of the patient to decide on the best timing for proceeding with transplantation. This approach is discussed further in Question 86 on page 181.

Radiation therapy can be another useful option for the treatment of indolent lymphoma. Very occasionally, patients may have stage I or II disease with one or two lymph node areas involved. In such cases, especially in the rare situation of stage I indolent lymphoma, radiation may actually provide a cure. If not a cure, it may actually delay the lymphoma from returning for many years.

Therapies for CLL/SLL utilize most of the same principles as other indolent lymphomas with a few variations. Based on well-designed trials, most physicians agree that FCR presently appears to be the most effective treatment for young fit patients with CLL who can tolerate what is a fairly aggressive treatment regimen. The combination of bendamustine and rituximab (BR) is also a very good regimen for many patients except perhaps for those with the highest risk genetics. Older fit patients can likely be treated safely with BR as well. For older patients who are less fit or who have other chronic illnesses, chemotherapy such as chlorambucil, or chlorambucil with a monoclonal antibody such as rituximab or more recently obinutuzumab or ofatumumab, are likely to be offered. Newer targeted therapies such as ibrutinib are making their way quickly into clinical practice. Ibrutinib is presently FDA approved for patients with CLL who have received at least one prior regimen for their illness. This is an oral medication taken daily for as long as it controls the illness and as long as there are no serious side effects. Unlike follicular lymphomas, autologous stem cell transplantation does not appear to be very effective in CLL. Allogeneic stem cell transplantation is feasible and may have curative potential in some individuals with CLL who are able to tolerate the therapy.

52. How does my doctor know what treatment to recommend for my indolent lymphoma?

Your lymphoma specialist will make a recommendation for treatment after reviewing all aspects of your particular lymphoma and your general state of health and your own preferences after you have an understanding of the various options available. Consideration of your general health and well-being is important in determining your ability to tolerate the different chemotherapy drugs or combination regimens and the optimal time for therapy to begin. Your doctor's experience in treating other patients with similar types of lymphoma, knowledge gained from reading the medical literature, continuing medical education (attending lectures or conferences), and discussions with colleagues all provide the background for making treatment recommendations. Many centers, especially the larger cancer centers, have a number of lymphoma specialists who discuss all of the new cases of lymphoma at a regular conference. Discussions from these tumor board meetings can be very helpful when deciding on a treatment plan. Pathologists and radiologists will often also be at this meeting; thus, all aspects of the case can be considered together. The discussion can also serve to provide you with a number of second opinions. There are also a number of online resources available to physicians with up-to-date treatment recommendations. Medical journal reviews are also very helpful.

It can be quite frustrating when your physician presents a number of different treatment options and suggests that you decide which option to proceed with. Given that many options may be right, you may need assistance with this decision; thus, you can ask your doctor for further guidance in making the best decision. Given that there are often a number of good treatment options with similar outcomes, understanding the pros and cons of each one will be helpful in allowing you to come to a decision on which one is right for you.

53. How are aggressive and highly aggressive lymphoma treated?

There are a number of lymphomas that are considered to be aggressive or highly aggressive because of their growth patterns or response to treatment. Examples of some common or characteristic disease entities are shown in **Table 13** on page 120.

These lymphomas are generally managed with the intent of treatment being a cure. The exception is mantle cell lymphoma, which, along with the indolent lymphomas, is generally considered to be incurable. As DLBCL-NOS is the most common of all lymphomas, it is discussed here in greatest detail.

The aggressive and highly aggressive lymphomas are frequently fast growing and require treatment soon after the diagnosis is made. Because many patients can be cured, the approach involves giving the treatment that is the most likely to result in a cure as the initial therapy. For many years, CHOP had been considered the best treatment for aggressive lymphomas such as DLBCL-NOS and, now, with the introduction of monoclonal antibodies such as rituximab, R-CHOP is now the most widely used treatment for these B-cell lymphomas. This is an outpatient treatment in most situations. Many similar chemotherapy regimens have been compared with CHOP, but in general, none have proven to be better. One potential exception to this is a regimen used in Europe known as ACVBP (doxorubicin, cyclophosphamide, vindesine, bleomycin, prednisone), which is given along with additional consolidation chemotherapy including methotrexate, ifosfamide, and cytarabine. Also, one of the chemotherapy agents in this regimen (vindesine) is not available in North America and therefore has not found its way into practice here. Before rituximab, overall, approximately 40–50% of patients were cured with the CHOP regimen. The IPI was helpful in determining this, but even a high IPI score did not exclude the possibility of cure, although the likelihood was lower. With rituximab, the results of therapy have significantly improved over the use of CHOP alone, even for patients with a higher IPI score. After the diagnosis and staging have been completed, most patients receive six to eight cycles of chemotherapy. R-CHOP is most commonly given every 3 weeks such that six cycles of chemotherapy can be delivered in 18 weeks if there are no treatment delays. Another regimen devised in the United States is

Table 13 Examples of Aggressive/Highly Aggressive Lymphomas

Diffuse large B-cell lymphoma
Follicular grade 3 lymphoma
Mantle cell lymphoma
Lymphoblastic lymphoma
Burkitt lymphoma
Peripheral T-cell lymphoma
Anaplastic large cell lymphoma
Adult T-cell leukemia/lymphoma

known as dose adjusted R-EPOCH (rituximab, etoposide, prednisone, vincristine, cyclophosphamide, doxorubicin). This regimen utilizes prolonged infusions of the chemotherapy agents and dose adjustments based on the blood counts during therapy to try to maximize the treatment effect. It is often used for aggressive and highly aggressive lymphomas and HIV-associated lymphomas. A randomized trial of R-EPOCH compared with R-CHOP for patients with newly diagnosed DLBCL is ongoing and initial results should be forthcoming within a short time.

Many investigators have tried to improve on the outcomes of aggressive lymphomas by adding additional treatment at the end of the initial chemotherapy. Although the concept of maintenance rituximab is attractive and beneficial in indolent lymphomas, it has not been shown to improve outcomes in aggressive lymphomas once they are in remission. Also the use of autologous **peripheral blood stem cell transplants** for patients in first remission has been looked at exhaustively in this patient population over the past 20 years or more. It is possible that some high-risk patients may receive some small additional gains from undergoing transplant in first remission, but this remains an area of controversy and is not considered a standard approach. Other maintenance strategies with newer agents are being explored in clinical trials. Also the newer targeted agents such as ibrutinib in combination with chemoimmunotherapy are being looked at in clinical trials of certain subsets of aggressive lymphomas.

For people whose lymphoma involves fewer lymph node areas (stage I or II with no bulky tumor masses), fewer cycles of therapy can safely be given. Essentially, only three cycles of R-CHOP need to be given, instead of

Peripheral blood stem cell transplant

A transplant using marrow stem cells that have been obtained from the blood circulation.

six to eight cycles, but only if radiation therapy is given to the one or two areas involved with the lymphoma. Studies have demonstrated that three cycles of chemotherapy followed by radiation are likely equivalent to six to eight cycles of chemotherapy in stage I or stage II aggressive lymphoma (e.g., DLBCL-NOS). Patients are therefore exposed to less chemotherapy, and the entire treatment course is shorter, potentially resulting in fewer complications from the treatment. Whether you can receive radiation and therefore be spared the extra cycles of chemotherapy depends on where the lymphoma is in your body. In some cases, it may be too risky to radiate particular areas of the body, and your doctor may prefer to administer six to eight cycles of chemotherapy.

Some patients, even though they receive six to eight cycles of chemotherapy, may still need radiation, especially if the site of lymphoma is bulky. Radiation to bulky sites that were present before chemotherapy, even if they have disappeared with treatment, may help prevent the lymphoma from returning at that site. Ongoing studies with the use of PET scans during or at the end of chemotherapy may help define a set of patients in whom additional treatment with radiation is not required.

54. How is HIV-associated lymphoma treated?

Treatment has dramatically improved since the introduction of HAART. These medications reduce the number and type of infections occurring during chemotherapy. Because of this, the doses of chemotherapy agents have been increased back to normal. Some of the HAART medications may need to be altered during chemotherapy. Your lymphoma doctor will want to know your current

HIV viral load and CD4 counts. Many things will come into consideration when deciding on the correct treatment. The exact type of lymphoma and its stage and your general health status are very important considerations. Chemotherapy will often be given along with monoclonal antibodies, as long as patients are not very immunosuppressed, based on lymphocyte counts. Monoclonal antibodies can frequently suppress humoral immunity, mediated by B-cells. Further immunosuppression can increase the risk of infections. Colony-stimulating growth factors may also be given. R-EPOCH is commonly used for aggressive HIV-associated lymphomas. A more intensive chemotherapy regimen such as R-CODOX-M/IVAC (rituximab, cyclophosophamide, vincristine, doxorubicin, methotrexate, ifosfamide, etoposide, cytarabine) may also be used for highly aggressive lymphomas such as Burkitt lymphoma.

55. Is aggressive and highly aggressive lymphoma curable if it returns after therapy or did not respond to therapy?

If your lymphoma either returns after chemotherapy or did not completely respond to therapy, a chance of cure is still possible. High-dose chemotherapy with an autologous stem cell transplant is the most accepted treatment for people in otherwise good general health. In order to determine whether patients are likely to respond to the high-dose chemotherapy and transplant, another chemotherapy regimen is first given to shrink the lymphoma. If the lymphoma responds to this treatment, a transplant is still a reasonable treatment option. Patients with aggressive lymphomas that do not enter remission with initial therapy should be referred to a transplant center, where a transplant physician can determine whether you are likely to derive benefit from the transplant and help coordinate the next chemotherapy regimen and timing of determination of remission. If a transplant is a possible option, a number of tests to evaluate your heart, kidney, and lung functions, as well as an assessment of your general ability to withstand the transplant will be required. These tests should be performed as you are receiving your chemotherapy so that there is no delay between the chemotherapy and the transplant. Of all patients who respond to the salvage chemotherapy and go on to receive an autologous transplant, approximately 35–40% may be cured. Patients who are not ultimately cured with this approach still may receive benefit in terms of experiencing a longer period of remission before the lymphoma returns. The chances of cure without a transplant in this setting are much smaller. The most common salvage chemotherapy regimens contain a class of chemotherapy drugs known as platinum compounds and are generally administered along with rituximab. They include the R-ESHAP, R-ICE (rituximab, etoposide, methylprednisolone, cytarabine, cisplatin; rituximab, ifosfamide, carboplatin, etoposide), and R-gemcitabine-oxaliplatin regimens, which are usually given two or three times at 2- to 4-week intervals depending on the regimen and the time to recovery of blood counts between cycles.

56. How is highly aggressive lymphoma treated?

In many cases, the highly aggressive lymphomas can also be cured with either chemotherapy alone or combined with monoclonal antibodies. These are generally very rapidly growing lymphomas, frequently resulting in the development of often bulky lymph nodes in a

In many cases, the highly aggressive lymphomas can also be cured with either chemotherapy alone or combined with monoclonal antibodies.

short period of time with the potential to cause obstruction of vital structures including the airway or nerve tissue, with the potential for paralysis. As a result, treatment is generally fairly urgent. The treatment regimens used for these lymphomas consist of a number of different chemotherapy drugs given at frequent intervals. Patients usually require hospitalization for the few days each month when the chemotherapy is administered. These regimens are similar to the treatments used for childhood leukemia. Because most of these lymphomas are very fast growing, they can also be very sensitive to the effects of chemotherapy; therefore, there is a very high rate of complete response. As a result of the often very rapid response, the lymph nodes can shrink very fast, often over a period of days. As the cancer cells die, they release a lot of different toxic substances into the bloodstream, which then have to be safely excreted from the body. The kidneys need to be functioning well to handle the extra workload, and extra measures need to be taken in preparation for the chemotherapy in an attempt to prevent serious problems, including kidney failure. Intravenous fluids are given in large quantities along with medications such as allopurinol or rasburicase. These measures help protect the kidneys and help the kidneys safely remove the products resulting from tumor cell death. The rapid production of these products of tumor cell death is known as tumor lysis. Tumor lysis is most common with highly aggressive lymphomas such as Burkitt lymphoma and lymphoblastic lymphoma. Even with proper precautions and correct use of fluids and medications like allopurinol, tumor lysis can still occasionally lead to some degree of kidney damage. In the most extreme cases significant kidney damage resulting in the need for dialysis may occur but this is almost always temporary and the kidneys generally recover normal or near normal function with time.

Once a remission is achieved, further cycles of therapy are given to prevent the lymphoma from returning. More cycles of the same or similar chemotherapy may be given. The number of cycles varies, as there are a number of different regimens available. If the lymphoma is a B-cell type and expresses CD20 on the surface of the lymphoma cells, monoclonal antibodies are given along with the chemotherapy.

An important aspect of treating high-grade lymphoma is treatment of the CNS. In certain circumstances and especially with highly aggressive lymphomas, the CNS may be involved at diagnosis or in the future with a recurrence. In these circumstances additional therapy is required to treat existing or prevent future CNS involvement. One means of evaluating and treating the CNS is to perform a **spinal tap** (lumbar puncture). The **spinal fluid** is analyzed for any lymphoma cells, and often, at the same time, a small amount of intrathecal chemotherapy is given through the spinal needle into the spinal fluid. The chemotherapy then circulates through the spinal fluid and the fluid around the brain. Giving this dose of chemotherapy even before knowing whether the lymphoma involves the CNS does no harm. If there is CNS lymphoma, more intrathecal chemotherapy and possibly radiation therapy or additional chemotherapy with high-dose intravenous methotrexate will be necessary. Even if there is no lymphoma present in the spinal fluid, most patients with highly aggressive lymphoma also need further intrathecal chemotherapy to prevent lymphoma from occurring at this site. Regimens designed for highly aggressive lymphomas generally include drugs such as methotrexate and cytarabine at doses substantial enough to allow the drugs to penetrate inside the CNS to some extent through the bloodstream.

Spinal tap

The procedure for obtaining a sample of spinal fluid.

Spinal fluid

The fluid surrounding the brain and spinal fluid.

In some patients, especially if the lymphoma recurs during or after a complete treatment course, an autologous stem cell transplant with high-dose chemotherapy may be considered and can result in a cure.

57. How is Hodgkin lymphoma treated?

Hodgkin lymphoma is, in a general sense, considered to be the most curable of all of the lymphomas. On average the cure rate is anywhere from 50–90%. In order to understand the treatment of Hodgkin lymphoma, it is important to realize that it tends to spread from one lymph node area to other lymph node areas close by as it progresses (i.e., in a somewhat orderly fashion). The non-Hodgkin lymphomas generally do not demonstrate this tendency; instead, they often skip areas. As a result, the stage of Hodgkin lymphoma is a very important factor in deciding on treatment. Another important factor is the type of Hodgkin lymphoma. There are two broad categories. The first is classical Hodgkin lymphoma, which includes the nodular sclerosis, mixed cellularity, lymphocyte-depleted and lymphocyte-rich types. The second is nodular lymphocyte–predominant Hodgkin lymphoma and it is often treated somewhat differently than classical Hodgkin lymphoma. It has features in common with indolent B-cell lymphomas. Another very important factor is whether the features at diagnosis are associated with a lower (favorable) or higher (unfavorable) risk of recurrence.

Before the availability of current imaging technology, physicians used to go to great lengths to determine the stage of the lymphoma. An operation called a staging laparotomy was performed if the lymphoma appeared to involve only one or two areas. This operation involved making an incision in the abdomen, taking small pieces (biopsies) of the liver and any lymph nodes, and also removing the spleen. This operation was done to be absolutely certain that the lymphoma was in only one or two areas. During the staging laparotomy era, patients with localized Hodgkin lymphoma were often treated with radiation alone. However, over time, it became clear that radiation treatment alone had its long-term drawbacks, and as such, combinations of chemotherapy and radiotherapy began to come into practice to limit the dose and size of the radiation field. With modern staging methods, staging laparotomy is virtually never performed today.

Currently, Hodgkin lymphoma that is stage I or stage II with favorable features (see Question 48 on page 106) is generally treated with both radiation and chemotherapy. Chemotherapy is given first and then followed by radiation. Sometimes, chemotherapy alone may be an alternative, and for patients unable to take any chemotherapy due to coexisting illnesses, radiation alone may be reasonable. For localized involvement of other areas, radiation alone was previously offered to most patients; however, some chemotherapy appears necessary in order to reduce the risk for relapse. Typically, four cycles of chemotherapy will be administered followed by radiation. Relatively recently, some newer data suggests that it may be possible to treat the very best subgroup of early-stage favorable patients with two cycles of chemotherapy followed by a smaller dose of radiation than is typically used, or four cycles of chemotherapy alone. For patients with stage I or II disease with unfavorable features, six cycles of chemotherapy will usually be given, and if any of the initial tumor sites were considered to be very large (bulky), generally radiation therapy will be delivered at the end of chemotherapy. The use of interim (i.e., performed part of the way through therapy) PET scans for Hodgkin lymphoma is becoming more accepted though data supporting their use to change treatment part way through therapy is limited in our opinion. The results of several ongoing clinical trials using this approach may further change some of these approaches in the coming few years.

For patients with stage III or IV disease, chemotherapy alone is the typical treatment, with radiation reserved for areas that may have been particularly bulky.

The most commonly used chemotherapy regimen in Hodgkin lymphoma is ABVD. This includes the drugs doxorubicin (Adriamycin®), bleomycin, vinblastine, and dacarbazine. Typically, six to eight cycles of therapy will be given, and each cycle consists of two treatments given every 2 weeks. This regimen is associated with fewer long-term side effects when compared to the older MOPP regimen. There is a much lower incidence of infertility and leukemia in later years. The MOPP regimen includes nitrogen mustard (mechlorethamine), vincristine (Oncovin®), prednisone, and procarbazine. The Stanford V regimen, pioneered at Stanford University, is a reasonable option for certain patients. This regimen administers all of the chemotherapy in 12 weeks, but all patients also generally need to receive radiation to involved sites. Chemotherapy is given weekly, and the drugs included in this regimen are nitrogen mustard, doxorubicin, vinblastine, vincristine, bleomycin, etoposide, and prednisone.

Another regimen that has been evaluated is the escalated BEACOPP regimen, developed in Germany. This regimen is often a compelling choice for young medically fit patients with early stage unfavorable disease or stage III or IV Hodgkin lymphoma with a higher number of risk factors according to the international prognostic score.

STAGING AND TREATMENT OF LYMPHOMA

The drugs included in this regimen are bleomycin, etoposide, doxorubicin (Adriamycin®), cyclophosphamide, vincristine (Oncovin®), procarbazine, and prednisone. This regimen has a considerably increased likelihood of side effects including the development of serious infections, but these may be warranted in patients who have a particularly high likelihood of recurrence.

Patients with Hodgkin lymphoma who are greater than 60 years of age constitute somewhat of a special situation. The results of treatment are generally not so optimistic in this group of patients. This is at least in part likely because they experience more side effects and frequently experience delays or require reductions in the doses of chemotherapy. For example bleomycin can be a more difficult agent to use safely in this age group because of an apparent increase in the risk of lung toxicity. The inferior outcomes may also be because the biology of Hodgkin lymphoma is different in older patients. In this age group a so-called hybrid regimen such as ChlVPP/ABV (chlorambucil, vinblastine, procarbazine, prednisone, doxorubicin, bleomycin, vincristine) or ChlVPP alone may be more tolerable. A medication known as brentuximab vedotin (see Question 58 on page 131) is now approved for patients with recurrent or refractory Hodgkin lymphoma, and this is being tested on its own, or in combination with some of the previously mentioned agents in clinical trials for people over 60 years of age to see if current treatment outcomes can be improved upon with a reduction in side-effects.

58. What happens if my Hodgkin lymphoma comes back?

Unfortunately, patients with Hodgkin lymphoma who achieve an initial complete remission may still experience a recurrence. The risk of recurrence can be estimated using the previously described prognostic features at the time of initial diagnosis. The prognostic scoring systems discussed in Question 48 on page 106 describe this in greater detail. The management of recurrent disease primarily depends on what treatment was previously given, the stage of the disease at the original diagnosis and at the time of recurrence, and the time interval between the original treatment and the recurrence. If the disease was limited and treated with radiation alone, most patients can receive one of the chemotherapy options discussed in the previous question with outcomes that are seemingly as good as newly diagnosed patients. Most patients, however, will have received chemotherapy previously. Such patients are generally considered candidates for high-dose chemotherapy and autologous stem cell transplantation, as discussed in Question 83 on page 175. If a long interval has elapsed between the original treatment and the recurrence, an alternative chemotherapy regimen or even possibly the same chemotherapy regimen as previously given may be considered, without including high-dose chemotherapy and autologous stem cell transplantation, although these situations are comparatively rare. The vast majority of relapsed patients are best treated with so-called salvage chemotherapy followed by autologous stem cell transplantation. It is important to realize that the healthiest and fittest older patients- including those who are in their seventh decade of life- may still be considered for autologous stem cell transplantation at some centers, as the long term outcomes with well selected patients may be nearly as good as those of younger patients.

Brentuximab vedotin is a monoclonal antibody directed against the cell surface protein known as CD30 that is expressed on the so-called Hodgkin Reed Sternberg cells. The antibody is linked (conjugated) to a chemotherapy agent known as monomethyl auristatin-E (MMAE). Brentuximab vedotin is approved for patients with relapsed or refractory Hodgkin lymphoma, and for patients with systemic anaplastic large cell lymphoma who have not entered remission after one line of chemotherapy. There are many clinical trials ongoing with this agent looking at its use in all common settings—as part of initial therapy, salvage therapy, or post autologous transplantation. The chemotherapy agent bendmustine has some activity in patients with Hodgkin lymphoma and is also being tested in various settings in Hodgkin lymphoma including in combination with brentuximab vedotin.

PART FOUR

Chemotherapy and Radiation Therapy

What is chemotherapy?

What chemotherapy drugs are used
to treat lymphoma?

How is chemotherapy given?

More . . .

59. What is chemotherapy?

Paul Erlich (1854–1915) introduced the concept of chemotherapy. His revolutionary idea was to use mice to test antibiotics for activity against infectious disease. Subsequently, mice with tumors were used to test the activity of other chemicals against cancer. Further advances in the development of chemotherapy were made during World War I. Mustard gas was being tested as a chemical weapon, and exposure to this agent led to shrinkage of lymph nodes and bone marrow. These observations led to the use of nitrogen mustard for the treatment of lymphoma in the early 1940s.

Chemotherapy actually means the treatment of disease with any drug. However, in common usage, it refers to the treatment of cancer using drugs. Chemotherapy drugs are the most widely used treatments for lymphoma. Many different types of chemotherapy drugs are available, and new ones are continuously being developed. Many are derived from natural products found in the environment. The National Cancer Institute has a specific program in which scientists all over the world obtain samples from plants, trees, ocean-dwelling creatures, and so forth, and test them in the laboratory for any activity against cancer.

Chemotherapy drugs are given orally or intravenously, or, less commonly, are injected directly into a muscle (**intramuscular**), under the skin (subcutaneous), or into the spinal fluid surrounding the brain and spinal cord (intrathecal). However the drugs are given, apart from intrathecally, the chemotherapy gets into the bloodstream and is distributed to all parts of the body. This type of treatment is referred to as **systemic treatment** and is different from **local treatment**, in which a specific

Intramuscular

An injection into the muscle.

Systemic treatment

A treatment, such as chemotherapy, that reaches all body parts through the bloodstream.

Local treatment

Treatment aimed at a particular area of the body. For example, radiation treatment is local, whereas chemotherapy is systemic.

site is targeted. Examples of local treatment include radiation and surgery. The benefit of chemotherapy over surgery or radiation is its ability to reach all parts of the lymphatic system. Depending on the specific type of lymphoma, even if lymph nodes in other areas are not enlarged, they may still be affected at the microscopic level and, therefore, benefit from chemotherapy. Surgery or radiation will not be helpful against these areas of microscopic involvement. Most chemotherapy drugs kill the more rapidly dividing cells. Lymphoma cells divide more rapidly than normal cells, especially the intermediate- and high-grade lymphomas. This explains their better response to chemotherapy than the indolent lymphomas. It also explains why chemotherapy affects the bone marrow, lining of the gut, and eggs and sperm more than slower dividing cells.

Chemotherapy drugs are classified into groups based on their exact mechanism of action on cell machinery. Different groups of drugs act at different phases of the cell life cycle. Drugs acting on different mechanisms within cancer cells are often used together as combination chemotherapy regimens, having a greater effect against the cancer than single drugs.

60. What conventional chemotherapy drugs are used to treat lymphoma?

The number of drugs available to treat lymphoma continues to increase. The oldest agents are commonly known as "conventional chemotherapy" or "conventional cytotoxic agents." These drugs work by getting inside lymphoma cells and causing damage generally to the DNA, to the enzymes that repair DNA, by interfering with new DNA synthesis or by interfering with cell division in other ways inside lymphoma cells. Many of them are highly effective at treating lymphoma, but nearly all have significant side effects because they cause similar damage to normal cells and organs (e.g., lungs, bone marrow, kidneys). This unwanted aspect of these agents generally limits the doses that can be given reasonably to the patient's cancer cells. Clinical studies continue to demonstrate better ways to use and combine chemotherapy drugs that have been available for many years. Chemotherapy drugs can be used either alone or in combination, and they are usually given orally as pills or intravenously. When given intravenously, they can be given as a **bolus** (a quick injection), short infusion, or continuous infusion (**Table 14**). Some of the general categories are discussed here.

Alkylating agents including chlorambucil and cyclophosphamide have been available for many years. Alkylating agents were the first chemotherapy drugs demonstrated to have anticancer activity in humans. During World War I, sulfur mustard gas was used as a weapon and was noted to produce **aplasia**, or shrinkage of lymph tissue. Subsequently, the related nitrogen mustards, which lacked the gases' nasty effects on the lungs and the skin, were examined for activity against lymphoma. Nitrogen mustard was developed as a result of such studies. Subsequently, other less toxic but more effective alkylating agents have been introduced. Chlorambucil and cyclophosphamide are currently the most commonly used alkylating agents that are used to treat lymphoma. Alkylating agents cause cross-linking of DNA, adding an extra chemical group to the DNA strands. This prevents the cell from dividing, which is necessary for its normal growth. Without the ability to divide, the cell dies.

Bolus

A rapid intravenous injection.

Alkylating agents

A class of chemotherapy drugs.

Aplasia

A condition where blood cells are not produced.

Chlorambucil and cyclophosphamide have been available for many years. Alkylating agents were the first chemotherapy drugs demonstrated to have anticancer activity in humans.

Chlorambucil is taken orally. There are many ways to dose this medication including 5-day periods every month, once every 2 weeks, or a lower dose given every day for a month at a time. It is generally well tolerated but can produce an upset stomach, which can be prevented with antinausea medication. It does not usually cause hair loss (**alopecia**). Its main side effect is to suppress the bone marrow, which is seen as a drop in the white blood cell count and the platelet count. Depending on how this medication is given, the maximum drop in the counts occurs at 3 to 4 weeks, and weekly counts are generally obtained to monitor the blood. Chlorambucil combined with prednisone may produce a slightly faster response than chlorambucil alone but does not have any other substantial benefit.

Alopecia
Hair loss.

Cyclophosphamide can be given intravenously or orally. For the treatment of indolent lymphoma, it is usually given orally as part of the CVP regimen, along with vincristine and prednisone, for 5 days every 3 weeks. It may cause some nausea and vomiting, which can be controlled with antinausea medicine, and frequently causes hair loss. When given over a prolonged period of time or in very large doses, it may cause bleeding from damage to the lining of the bladder. Cyclophosphamide also affects the blood counts. A drop in the white blood cell count is usually seen (greatest at 10 to 14 days).

An important consideration when taking alkylating agents is the risk of second cancers. These may develop years after receiving these agents. The risk for developing leukemia is estimated at approximately 6% and emphasizes the need to consider possible long-term complications of any treatment, especially for somebody without symptoms.

CHEMOTHERAPY AND RADIATION THERAPY

Antitumor antibiotics

A class of chemotherapy drugs.

Another class of chemotherapy drugs commonly used for the treatment of lymphoma are **antitumor antibiotics**. Doxorubicin belongs to this class of drugs, and it causes cancer cells to die by interfering with the DNA. Mitoxantrone is a similar drug. Doxorubicin is generally combined with cyclophosphamide, vincristine, and prednisone in the CHOP regimen. If mitoxantrone is used instead of doxorubicin, it is called **CNOP**. CHOP is the most commonly used regimen for the aggressive lymphomas but is also frequently used as a treatment option for indolent lymphomas. It is generally administered every 3 weeks for six to eight cycles.

CNOP

A combination chemotherapy regimen.

Side effects of doxorubicin also include bone marrow suppression. The lowest blood counts are at 10 to 14 days. Nausea and vomiting are usually preventable with premedication, and hair loss also occurs. Doxorubicin can also occasionally produce heart muscle damage and with prolonged treatment, may even produce heart failure. Because of this small risk, a measurement of heart function is often obtained before starting the CHOP regimen. As initial therapy for indolent lymphoma, CHOP does not appear to be better than chlorambucil or CVP in terms of lengthening overall years of life, but it produces a more rapid response and maybe a higher chance of a complete response. In certain cases, it may offer significant advantages over other treatments.

Nucleoside analogues

A type of chemotherapy drug that targets lymphocytes.

Another class of drugs used to treat lymphoma is **nucleoside analogues**. Fludarabine is an example of this type of drug. Fludarabine is taken up into lymphocytes and blocks the activity of an enzyme important for lymphocyte growth. It is quite active against cells that divide only slowly, including the indolent lymphomas.

Fludarabine is given as an intravenous infusion over 30 minutes, generally for 3-5 days in a row every month (each cycle lasting for 1 month) for a variable number of cycles, depending on how well the patient responds. Some nausea or vomiting may occur but is unusual. Bone marrow suppression occurs, resulting in the need to monitor blood counts regularly. Fludarabine is also quite effective at killing normal lymphocytes, and this can be a very long-lasting effect. As a result, patients are at higher risk of developing certain infections such as **shingles** or even *Pneumocystis jarovecii pneumonia*, an infection more commonly seen in individuals with uncontrolled HIV infection. The antibiotic trimethoprim-sulfamethoxazole is very effective at preventing this infection when given twice a week.

Fludarabine has been administered in combination with other chemotherapy drugs such as cyclophosphamide and mitoxantrone. The combination may have advantages in certain individuals, but the incidence of side effects is greater.

Vincristine and vinblastine belong to a class of drugs called the **vinca alkaloids**. The vinca alkaloids inhibit cancer cells by binding to **microtubules**, which prevent the cell from dividing normally. Both drugs are given intravenously and usually are part of a combination chemotherapy regimen. Vincristine is the *V* in the CVP regimen and also the *O* in the CHOP regimen. Vinblastine is more commonly used in the treatment of Hodgkin lymphoma.

Hair loss may occur with both drugs, although more commonly with vincristine. The main side effect of vincristine is mild nerve damage, referred to as peripheral neuropathy. This is quite common, and the frequency

Shingles

A painful condition with a rash, usually affecting one area of the skin in the distribution of a nerve. It is due to reactivation of the chickenpox virus and usually occurs when the immune system is depressed.

Pneumocystis jarovecii pneumoniae

An infection affecting the lungs that can occur in people with an abnormal immune system.

Vinca alkaloids

A type of chemotherapy drug.

Microtubules

Structures present in individual cells that are important for allowing cells to divide.

increases with ongoing treatment. Often the first thing noticed is tingling in the fingers and toes. It is important at clinic visits to tell your physician about these changes. Jaw pain may also occur because the drug affects nerves in that area. Constipation as a result of vincristine affecting the nerves of the gut is also common, and, if necessary, you should take a stool softener or a laxative to try and prevent and manage this complication. The nerve damage that vincristine causes is generally reversible but may take many months to return to normal. Your doctor may reduce the dose or stop the drug completely, depending on your symptoms, which generally improve after the drug is discontinued.

Etoposide kills lymphoma cells by interacting with a protein that is important for stabilizing DNA.

Ifosfamide and carboplatin are active in lymphoma. These drugs are often used together with etoposide in the ICE regimen. Ifosfamide belongs to the same class as cyclophosphamide and has a similar side effect profile. Carboplatin is a similar drug to cisplatinum, but its main side effect is bone marrow suppression.

61. How is chemotherapy given?

Most patients with lymphoma receive chemotherapy intravenously. Other ways to administer the drugs include by mouth, under the skin, into the muscle, or into the CSF (intrathecally).

Indwelling catheter

An intravenous catheter that can remain in place for longer than a few days.

If a number of cycles of chemotherapy are to be given intravenously, one potentially very useful item is an **indwelling catheter**. Having a catheter can simplify the process of receiving chemotherapy infusions or injections

Table 14 Standard Chemotherapy Regimens for Lymphoma

Chemotherapy drugs and combinations	How given
Bendamustine	Intravenously
Chlorambucil with or without prednisone	Orally or intravenously
Cyclophosphamide (C)	Orally
Vincristine (O or V)	Intravenously
Prednisone (P)	Orally
Fludarabine	Intravenously
Cyclophosphamide (C)	Intravenously
Doxorubicin (H)	Intravenously
Vincristine (O)	Intravenously
Prednisone (P)	Orally
Fludarabine (F)	Intravenously
Cyclophosphamide (C)	Intravenously
Fludarabine (F)	Intravenously
Mitoxantrone (N)	Intravenously
Dexamethasone (D)	Intravenously
Cyclophosphamide (C)	Intravenously
Mitoxantrone (N)	Intravenously
Vincristine (O)	Intravenously
Prednisone (P)	Orally
Ifosfamide (I)	Intravenously
Carboplatin (C)	Intravenously
Etoposide (E)	Intravenously
Etoposide (E)	Intravenously
Solumedrol (S)	Intravenously
Ara-C (HA)	Intravenously
Cisplatinum (P)	Intravenously
Rituximab (R)	Intravenously
Rituximab + CHOP	Intravenously
Rituximab + other chemotherapy	Intravenously

and can decrease the chances of substantial inflammation of the veins (phlebitis) associated with many chemotherapy drugs. Indwelling catheters are essentially hollow tubes, one end of which is placed into a vein close to the heart. The other end of the tube is conveniently located under the skin or actually comes out through the skin, where it is available for connection to the chemotherapy bag. This prevents needing to find a vein and inserting a new intravenous needle each time that chemotherapy is given. It is also a safer way to administer chemotherapy. The catheters are also useful for taking blood samples. Blood transfusions, antibiotics, or intravenous fluids can also be given through the catheter.

Several different types of indwelling catheters exist and can remain in place for many months or even a year or more. Two main styles of catheter exist and differ depending on whether they are implanted entirely under the skin, as in the case of the **Portacath**, or whether a part of the catheter comes out through the skin (**Figure 3**).

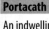

Portacath

An indwelling intravenous catheter that is placed entirely underneath the skin.

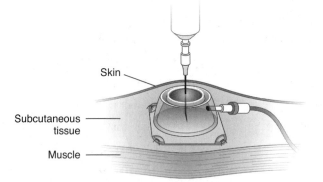

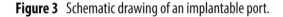

Figure 3 Schematic drawing of an implantable port.

The first type of catheter is a **Hickman** or **Broviac catheter**. Part of it is external, with approximately 6 inches of tubing outside the skin. This catheter requires dressing changes, and the tubes need to be flushed daily with a medication to keep blood from clotting in it. The patient can be taught to do this at home. The second type of catheter is a port or Portacath (Figure 3), which remains entirely under the skin without any external component. It does not require any dressing and requires only monthly flushing. The flushing requires the services of a nurse, and each time the port is accessed, it requires that a needle be inserted through the skin. In the case of both catheters, the part that is accessed for chemotherapy is usually placed on the upper part of the chest. Smaller catheters may also be useful in some situations and may be placed in the arms instead of the chest wall, such as the percutaneous implantable central catheter (PICC; **Figure 4**).

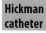

Hickman catheter

An intravenous line that passes through the skin into a large vein near the heart. It provides a safer and easier way to administer chemotherapy and obtain blood samples.

Broviac catheter

A type of catheter that goes directly into a large vein to allow easier administration of medications and blood tests.

CHEMOTHERAPY AND RADIATION THERAPY

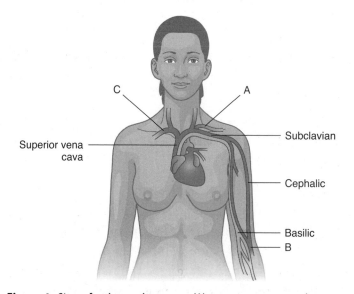

Superior vena cava
Subclavian
Cephalic
Basilic

Figure 4 Sites of catheter placement: (A) percutaneous central venous catheters; (B) PICC lines; (C) can be in the subclavian vein on either side; the access for the catheter is usually placed in the upper chest wall and tunnelled under the skin to the point of insertion into the vein.

62. What problems can result from having a catheter?

Side effects from catheters do occur, but in most patients, the convenience and comfort of a catheter outweigh its risks. A surgeon or an **interventional radiologist** (a doctor who performs surgical procedures such as placing an intravenous catheter using X-ray equipment) places these catheters, usually using local anesthesia. Complications rarely occur at the time that a catheter is first placed but include bleeding that is usually easily controlled. More seriously, but quite rarely, a lung can be punctured. Symptoms of a punctured lung include shortness of breath, cough, and chest pain. If there is any doubt, your doctor will obtain a chest X-ray.

Complications that may develop during the time a catheter is in place can include infection or a blood clot forming around the catheter.

If you want an indwelling catheter and your healthcare team recommends this approach, you can discuss which catheter is most appropriate.

Interventional radiologist

A physician who is trained in using X-rays to aid in the performance of some types of surgical procedures.

Side effects from catheters do occur, but in most patients, the convenience and comfort of a catheter outweigh its risks.

63. What are the side effects of chemotherapy?

In this question, we discuss general side effects that may occur with most chemotherapy drugs. The extent of side effects varies depending on the specific drugs that you receive, how they are administered, and how your body reacts to them. Your doctor and nurse will explain the side effects that you are most likely to experience. Most people associate nausea, vomiting, and hair loss with chemotherapy, but this is variable from person to person depending on the chemotherapy regimen. Today, good drugs are available to prevent nausea and vomiting. Thus, if you experience nausea or vomiting the first time that you receive chemotherapy, ask your physician whether any changes can be made for future treatments.

Most chemotherapy drugs kill some normal cells as well as lymphoma cells. Some of the side effects that you experience result from damage to these normal cells. The normal cells that are the most affected are those in areas where cells grow and divide most rapidly. These areas include hair follicles, bone marrow, the gastrointestinal tract, and the **reproductive system**. Thus, the most common side effects are hair loss, mouth sores, diarrhea, and problems related to infertility, although you should remember that having had chemotherapy does not necessarily mean that you are infertile. Because most chemotherapy drugs have severe effects on sperm and eggs, it is very important not to conceive while receiving chemotherapy. Appropriate contraception practices should be used if there is any potential for pregnancy.

Reproductive system

The body parts associated with reproduction.

64. Will I lose my hair?

Many patients undergoing chemotherapy are understandably anxious about hair loss. Your doctor and nurse will discuss the likelihood of this in your case. The likelihood of hair loss and how much to expect depends on the type of chemotherapy drugs that you receive, how frequently they are given, and the duration of treatment. For many patients, especially women, hair loss can be the most traumatic part of the entire treatment process. Loss of hair is a very obvious change in your appearance and can understandably have a considerable affect

The hair loss associated with chemotherapy usually begins 2 to 4 weeks after your treatment has begun. It is usually temporary and grows back starting 1 to 2 months after the completion of therapy.

on self-esteem. It may be the most visible sign that there is a problem. It can occur in other areas apart from the scalp. A loss of facial hair (eyebrows, eyelashes, mustache, and beard), axillary (underarm) hair, and pubic hair occurs with the longer chemotherapy regimens. The hair loss can vary, with some people experiencing thinning and others experiencing complete hair loss. The hair loss associated with chemotherapy usually begins 2 to 4 weeks after your treatment has begun. It is usually temporary and grows back starting 1 to 2 months after the completion of therapy. Your new hair may have a different texture or color; for example, it may grow back curly, whereas before chemotherapy it was straight.

65. How can I cope with hair loss?

First, discuss hair loss with your physician and nurse, your close family members, and/or your friends. You may wish to purchase a wig before your first treatment begins so that the color and texture can be closely matched to your own hair color. Many patients prefer to wear a head-scarf or bandana rather than a wig, whereas others prefer no head covering. The best thing to do is whatever feels right to you. The American Cancer Society offers an entire program that addresses hair loss and how it affects your appearance. The program is called "Look Good, Feel Better," and it offers seminars as well as one-on-one appointments with professional hair stylists and makeup artists. It offers fashion tips for wearing scarves as well as wigs. Information about this program is available from the American Cancer Society through a toll-free number (1-800-395-LOOK) that operates 24 hours a day, 7 days a week. The American Cancer Society also offers wigs that are free of charge, and some insurance companies will cover the cost of wigs. Otherwise, the cost should be tax deductible.

66. Will I have nausea and vomiting with treatment?

Years ago, patients receiving chemotherapy may have gotten very sick and experienced much vomiting. Today, however, there are many more chemotherapy drugs and other treatments that do not cause significant nausea and/or vomiting. In addition, there are several newer antinausea (**antiemetic**) medications that are very effective in preventing this problem. If necessary, your physician will prescribe antinausea drugs along with your chemotherapy. If you are still having nausea or vomiting, inform your doctor or nurse so that they can alter your antinausea drug regimen. Do not assume that you have to tough it out. Also, because everybody responds differently to different regimens, the first antinausea regimen may not work well for you, and alternatives are available. Sometimes a small dose of a steroid can be beneficial when added to other antinausea medications.

Also, rather than eating regular-sized meals, eating several smaller meals throughout the day can be helpful. You should avoid fried or fatty foods and should eat and drink slowly. Although rest is also helpful after a meal, you should not lie flat for at least 2 hours after eating.

Antiemetic
A medication to prevent nausea and vomiting.

67. Do I need to change my diet?

Good nutrition, although frequently neglected in the American diet, is always important. The same applies, even more so, as you proceed in your fight against lymphoma. What good nutrition means will vary according to your specific circumstances. Consulting with a dietician can be helpful. Eating adequate amounts of a healthy diet may help you feel better in general. When your body is receiving all that it needs, your ability to tolerate the side effects of the lymphoma may be improved, and you may also decrease your chance of infection through a beneficial effect on the immune system. A healthy diet and good nutrition will enhance your ability to maintain your strength and energy level, counteracting fatigue.

For those of you who do not have any specific problems that interfere with your appetite or ability to eat, we suggest that you follow the guidelines set by the U.S. Department of Agriculture, which outline what to eat on a daily basis (www.cnpp.usda.gov/dietaryguidelines.htm). Use this as a rough guide, possibly adding one to two servings from the milk group and one to two servings from the meat group. This will increase your total protein intake, which often is needed during an illness.

Changing your diet is a relatively easy step to take and is an aspect of your health in which you can have direct control. This is important at a time when you may feel that so many things fall outside of your control. Making your diet healthier may carry the benefits discussed previously, but as far as we know will not directly treat the lymphoma. Even the National Cancer Institute's stance is that there is not any evidence that any specific kind of diet or food alone can either cure cancer or keep it from coming back.

If you have lost weight, you may be able to focus on increasing your protein and energy (caloric) intake. If your appetite is good, this is fairly easy to accomplish. Focus on eating more high-calorie foods that provide protein, such as milk, cheese, and eggs. Sauces and gravies are also an efficient way of obtaining more calories.

If your appetite is poor, the same high-calorie and high-protein diet is encouraged. Try to eat several (five or six) small meals throughout the day and to include high-protein snacks such as ice cream, pudding, cheese, and peanut butter. At those times when you are not able to face a meal, a nourishing drink is an acceptable alternative. You can also add these drinks between meals to help with weight gain.

Several different commercially available supplements can add calories and protein to your diet. These taste best when served very cold. If the taste of one brand or flavor does not appeal to you, try another. Many people doctor up these drinks; for example, if the chocolate variety is too chocolaty or too sweet, try mixing it in a blender with some milk or vanilla ice cream. Alternatively, try adding some fruit, milk, or other flavor of ice cream to a vanilla variety drink. You can also create a milk shake from scratch. Or, combine milk with various fruits or fruit yogurt to make a smoothie. You can also add a scoop of ice cream and a few teaspoons of protein powder. Although these powders are commonly available, you should consult your healthcare team before using any dietary supplements.

At times you may want some foods that may be considered unhealthy. You may need to eat whatever food you can to obtain enough calories. Sometimes you may need to think of food like medicine: take some every 2 to 3 hours whether you feel like it or not. Be conscious of what you are eating, but, on the other hand, do not become obsessed. Mealtimes should be enjoyable and not a source of stress.

If you do not feel like preparing a meal, frozen dinners and microwaveable foods are convenient. This is also a perfect opportunity to give family and friends the chance to help you (e.g., going to the grocery store

CHEMOTHERAPY AND RADIATION THERAPY

or doing some cooking). If you have times when your energy level is better and you enjoy cooking, you could prepare some meals in advance and freeze them for later. If you really cannot face preparing or eating a meal, have one of the nutritional supplements discussed previously. Of course, eating out is an alternative. At certain times during chemotherapy, especially when your white blood cell count is low, you may be restricted to a **low microbial diet**—one that limits your exposure to foodborne bacteria or fungi.

Low microbial diet

A diet that that limits your exposure to food-borne bacteria or fungi.

68. What should I do if I'm having side effects that interfere with eating?

A sore throat or mouth sores from chemotherapy or radiation can result in difficulty eating. Crunchy foods such as raw fruits and vegetables, dry breads and cereals, spicy foods, and citrus should be avoided. Instead, eat soft and creamy food such as yogurt, pudding, buttered noodles, and cooked cereal. You may also find that foods that are too hot can also cause discomfort. Lukewarm or cool foods tend to be more soothing.

If you cannot tolerate solids, try liquid foods such as cream soups or nutrition drinks and shakes.

If nausea or vomiting is a problem, try sipping fluids throughout the day (along with trying antinausea medications), because you need to drink enough fluids to prevent dehydration.

If nausea or vomiting is a problem, try sipping fluids throughout the day (along with trying antinausea medications), because you need to drink enough fluids to prevent dehydration. Water is good, but juice-type commercial supplements may be even better. These provide protein as well as calories.

If you're feeling queasy but are not vomiting, try eating bland foods that are easy to digest (e.g., crackers, toast, rice, gelatin, and sherbet). These foods are not adequate sources of protein, calories, or nutrients, but this diet can be followed for a few days until the nausea subsides, as long as you are drinking enough liquids.

Sometimes food that you have previously enjoyed may taste bland. This can be the result of various medications, including chemotherapy. This change in taste may result in a loss of appetite and a failure to obtain adequate nutrition. Again, treating food like medicine—eating small amounts at regular intervals—may be a way to overcome this problem. You may need to experiment with new foods or new seasonings, or may need to add additional sugar, salt, or other flavor to enhance the taste. Most people report that cold or room-temperature foods are less offensive in their smell and taste.

If you simply have no appetite (**anorexia**), you may benefit from **megestrol acetate** (Megace), which is a hormonal agent that can stimulate the appetite and result in a weight gain. This is an option that you should discuss with your physician.

Anorexia
Loss of appetite.

Megestrol acetate
A medication that can increase the appetite.

69. How do I cope with anemia?

Anemia is common in patients with lymphoma. A blood test measures the hemoglobin level, or the **hematocrit**. Symptoms of anemia include fatigue, weakness, shortness of breath, headache, ringing in the ears, **palpitations** (an increased awareness of the heart beating), nausea, and occasional chest pain.

Hematocrit
A measure of the number of red cells, useful for anemia or polycythemia (too many red cells).

Palpitations
The sensation of an irregular heartbeat.

Anemia can occur for many different reasons. Often, bone marrow reacts to lymphoma in your body by decreasing the production of red blood cells. This also happens in people with many other illnesses, not just cancer. It occurs with infections and arthritis. This type of anemia is called **anemia of chronic disease**.

Anemia of chronic disease

Anemia caused by the bone marrow's reaction to being sick.

Lymphoma involving the bone marrow can also cause anemia. Bleeding can obviously lead to anemia and also needs to be considered as a cause. If bleeding occurs, report it to your physician. Having black, tarry bowel movements is a sign of bleeding in the bowels and requires urgent attention.

Chemotherapy commonly causes or worsens anemia and may contribute to fatigue (Question 72 on page 157). You should note that anemia is only one of many factors that contribute to fatigue.

Your doctor may perform tests to determine the reasons for the anemia. Deficiencies of iron, vitamin B_{12}, or folic acid are possible causes that simple blood tests can easily evaluate. If any of these are deficient, supplements can be provided. More commonly, anemia is not due to any deficiency in your diet and is therefore unlikely to respond to dietary supplements. Question 72 on page 157 discusses the use of **erythropoietin** in preventing or treating anemia.

Erythropoietin

A hormone produced by the kidneys that stimulates the bone marrow to produce red blood cells.

When you have symptoms from anemia, you should not overdo activities. Exercising is generally a good thing and should be encouraged but not pushed too hard. Limiting your activities to what you feel up to and getting plenty of rest can help to improve your sense of well-being.

70. Why is having a low white blood count such a concern?

Another common effect of chemotherapy is the reduction of the white blood cell count (**neutropenia**), which increases the risk of developing an infection. Although it seems like reasonable advice to tell patients to avoid large crowds, particularly during cold and flu season, there is no real data to substantiate the benefit of doing this. It is important to understand that the most common infections during periods of a low blood count actually arise from sources of bacteria within your own body. The probability of developing an infection is higher in older patients and in those with other medical problems such as chronic lung disease or diabetes. Having a central venous catheter may also slightly increase the chance of developing an infection. Even if you take precautions, infections are not entirely preventable. The risk of infection is highest with lower white blood cell counts and is also related to longer durations of neutropenia. Certain chemotherapy drugs or combinations of drugs are associated with a higher risk of infections than others.

If a fever develops while you are receiving chemotherapy or in the period afterward when your white count is low, you should seek medical attention without delay, especially if it is above 100.5°F. With neutropenia, infections can progress very rapidly and can even result in death if antibiotics are not started promptly. Patients are generally given very explicit instructions about dealing with fever or other infectious symptoms, and are often given cards to carry to present to an emergency room physician to assist with rapid evaluation and treatment of a fever. Cultures of blood and urine will usually be taken prior to rapidly starting an antibiotic. If the infection is bacterial these cultures may help determine the

Neutropenia

A low level of neutrophils.

organism causing the infection. A chest X-ray will usually also be taken to see if a pneumonia is the cause of the fever.

The development of a fever may require a hospital admission. For this reason, it is a good idea to keep a weekend bag packed. Sometimes, after the fever is assessed, an outpatient antibiotic treatment may be adequate.

Depending on the chemotherapy that you receive and on other factors such as your age and general health, your physician may prescribe a white blood cell growth factor in an effort to help your white blood cell count to recover sooner after chemotherapy. Most commonly, granulocyte-colony stimulating factor (G-CSF; Neupogen®), is used for this purpose. It is administered by a daily subcutaneous injection until the white blood cell count has recovered. A chemically altered version of Neupogen called Neulasta® remains in the circulation for a considerably longer period of time until the white blood cell count recovers and therefore only needs to be given once with every chemotherapy cycle. Like Neupogen®, Neulasta® is given as a subcutaneous injection.

Not everybody on chemotherapy needs to get a white blood cell growth factor. The decision is based on how likely you are to get an infection while on chemotherapy and whether you have previously experienced an infection. Discuss the need for a growth factor with your physician. The American Society of Clinical Oncology has developed guidelines for when these growth factors should be administered.

71. How do lymphoma and its treatment affect my sexuality?

It is not uncommon for lymphoma and its treatment to bring about physical and/or emotional changes that affect your sexual relationship. The degree to which this occurs depends on several factors, including the stage and symptoms of your lymphoma and the treatment that you are undergoing, as well as your overall emotional state.

It is difficult for some people to initiate conversations about sexuality with their partner; however, it can be very beneficial to speak openly and honestly with each other about your needs and wants. If you cannot do this, you might find it helpful to see a counselor or therapist on a short-term basis.

Although it may be even harder to discuss sexuality with strangers, a discussion with your healthcare team may help you to adjust to any changes as they occur. If your doctor or nurse is not helpful, speaking to the social worker may be beneficial.

One common issue that you may face as a result of your lymphoma and your treatment is a decreased sex drive, which can be a direct effect of your treatment or associated with fatigue or stress. It is important that this does not become the cause of further stress in your relationship. With good communication, your partner should understand the reasons for the decreased **libido**. You can also remind your partner that this is a temporary disruption, and once treatment (or the fatigue associated with it) is over, your sex drive will return to its former level. Depression, which is treatable, should also be considered as a possible cause for decreased libido.

Libido
Sex drive.

CHEMOTHERAPY AND RADIATION THERAPY

Chemotherapy and radiation can cause dryness of a woman's vagina. A water-soluble lubricant can help ease discomfort associated with decreased vaginal lubrication. Also, keep an open mind that there are different ways to feel sexual pleasure, as there may be times when intercourse is not possible. It is very important that you and your partner continue other ways of expressing affection for each other. Sometimes just cuddling can be enough, or you may want to explore other ways of caressing and stimulating each other.

Testosterone

A male hormone.

Chemotherapy and radiation can also result in low **testosterone** levels, which result in difficulty obtaining or maintaining an erection. Replacing testosterone may be all that is required. Sometimes antidepressants may interfere with a man's ability to function during intercourse.

Lymphoma cannot be passed through sexual intercourse. However, small amounts of chemotherapy can be present in semen of men receiving treatment, so condoms are highly recommended. People who have had a stem cell transplant should discuss the need to use condoms with their physicians.

Some people choose to wait to focus on the sexual part of their relationship until treatment is complete. Only you and your partner can decide what is best. Honesty and open communication avoid hurt feelings and misunderstandings and are an important part of resuming normal sexual activity.

72. Is fatigue always due to chemotherapy?

Fatigue, a very common symptom for many patients with cancer, can vary from slight fatigue, making everyday activities slightly more burdensome, to profound fatigue, resulting in extreme difficulty even getting out of bed. Fatigue can be extremely incapacitating, resulting in major impairment in quality of life, and is common even in patients who are not receiving chemotherapy. Many causes of fatigue exist among cancer patients, with anemia being one. This may be related to lymphoma's bone marrow involvement, resulting in decreased red blood cell production. Even without bone marrow involvement, anemia of chronic disease may also be present and may contribute to fatigue, which cytokine production can cause. Cytokines are chemicals that tumor cells produce in response to an infection. Lymphoma patients are understandably under a lot of stress, which is another cause of fatigue. Depression can add to the fatigue. Medications should also be evaluated as an additional factor that contributes to stress.

Discuss fatigue with your physician or nurse if it is an issue. If anemia is a significant component causing fatigue, a blood transfusion may be necessary. Erythropoietin is a hormone that is available for injection and may be beneficial in some circumstances (the kidneys produce erythropoietin, which then travels to the bone marrow cells and stimulates the production of red blood cells). It is available as a medication in a number of different preparations and is given by a subcutaneous or intravenous injection. It has been used for many years and is very similar to the naturally produced erythropoietin that the kidneys produce. It can be given either three times per week or once per week. Another

CHEMOTHERAPY AND RADIATION THERAPY

version that is long-acting, darbepoietin alpha, can be given every 2 weeks and appears to be similarly effective. Because there are many other causes of fatigue besides anemia, erythropoietin will not benefit all patients. With these medications, there is evidence of an increased risk of blood clots, heart attacks, strokes and even an increased risk of death and this should be discussed with your physician. Your list of medications should also be evaluated. If any medications can be discontinued, this may be helpful. Again, discuss this with your physician.

Maintaining a good caloric intake and adequate hydration is also important in counteracting fatigue. Plan your daily activities with an emphasis on the activities that are more important. It is quite acceptable to take naps, but sleeping too much during the day can further disrupt your sleeping pattern. Some daily exercise as tolerated can also be helpful in managing your fatigue.

73. Does chemotherapy cause bleeding?

Chemotherapy may cause bleeding, which is generally due to a fall in the platelet count. Depending on the type of chemotherapy you receive, regular blood counts may be important to obtain while you are receiving chemotherapy and will help to detect the need for platelet transfusions. If you develop any abnormal bleeding while on chemotherapy, inform your doctor. Abnormal bruising in addition to bleeding is also important. Other signs of a low platelet count include **petechiae**, which are small, purple, reddish spots on your skin that are actually tiny areas of bleeding generally around the hair follicles. They are most frequently seen on the front of your shins. During periods when your platelet count is

Petechiae

Pinpoint red spots that occur with low platelet counts and are due to tiny areas of bleeding into the skin.

low, you should avoid razor blades for shaving (use electric razors instead), nail clippers, and dental floss. For mouth care, you should use only a very soft toothbrush or sponges.

The occurrence of low platelet counts during chemotherapy depends on a number of factors, including the type of chemotherapy being administered, the amount of chemotherapy that the patient has previously received, and whether and to what degree the bone marrow is involved with lymphoma. It is important to control any existing high blood pressure when the platelet count is low, as the risk of bleeding may be increased.

Activities such as contact sports that could result in trauma need to be curtailed while the platelet count is low. Discuss any such activities with your physician before participation.

74. What is radiation therapy?

Radiation therapy uses high-energy X-rays to kill or prevent cancer cells from growing. Cancer cells grow faster than normal cells, so they are more susceptible to radiation. Because radiation therapy can also damage normal tissues around the area being radiated, a treatment plan is made to minimize the dose of radiation received by nearby normal tissues. This plan is generated by performing a **simulation**, at which time tiny tattoo marks or dots will be placed on your skin to mark the area to be radiated. Areas that are not to receive radiation will be protected with lead shielding. The radiation treatment itself takes only a few minutes, but treatment is spread over a few days to a few weeks, depending on the total dose of radiation to be administered. For treatment, you

Radiation therapy uses high-energy X-rays to kill or prevent cancer cells from growing.

Simulation

The planning necessary before administering any radiation treatment.

will generally be lying on a table close to a noisy radiation machine.

Before starting radiation treatment, you will have an appointment with a radiation oncologist, who specializes in radiation therapy to treat cancer. At the initial visit, your case will be reviewed to ensure that you are to benefit from radiation treatment and that the treatment can be given safely. The radiation oncologist will also review any scans or X-ray tests, as these will be helpful for planning the exact area that needs radiation. After this visit, you should have a good understanding of the reasons for needing radiation treatment, what to expect from the radiation in terms of side effects, and how long the treatment course will be.

Radiation is referred to as local treatment, being useful when treating particular sites within the body. The field of treatment is called a radiation port. **Total body irradiation** refers to the radiation of the whole body and is sometimes used in preparation for a stem cell transplant.

Total body irradiation

Radiation therapy administered to the entire body, usually in preparation for a transplant.

75. Will I need radiation therapy?

Radiation therapy can be useful for the treatment of lymphoma under many different circumstances. It may be used on its own in certain situations, or may be used to allow the number of chemotherapy cycles to be decreased (e.g., for some stage I or II lymphomas), or it may be used at the end of a full course of chemotherapy to treat areas of lymphoma that were very large at diagnosis or relapse

Radiation can rapidly control lymphoma at specific sites if necessary. An example of such a need is pain control due to lymphoma growing at one site or lymphoma pressing on the spinal cord, causing nerve damage. Spinal cord compression is a very urgent situation in which the lymphoma presses on the spinal cord, causing weakness (often in the legs), numbness, and possible loss of control of bladder or bowel function. These symptoms require extremely urgent medical attention because unless they are corrected rapidly, the nerve damage may be permanent.

76. What are the side effects of radiation therapy?

Radiation therapy itself is painless and does not cause you to become radioactive; however, you may experience some side effects depending on the part of your body that is being radiated. Other factors include the dose of radiation and whether chemotherapy is given at the same time. Side effects may be localized to the body part being treated or can be more widespread. Be sure to report any and all side effects to your healthcare team, as most can be effectively managed. Also remember that although side effects can be unpleasant, most are temporary and will gradually disappear after the treatment is finished.

During radiation therapy, the skin in the area being treated may become dry, irritated, and sensitive; it may feel and look sunburned and may also become itchy and then peel. To avoid further irritation, radiated areas should be kept clean using only warm water and very mild cleansers. Your healthcare team may prescribe or recommend creams, lotions, or ointments. You should avoid all cosmetics, deodorants, perfumes, powders, and other products that increase irritation in the affected area and that your healthcare team has not approved. It is also important to avoid sun exposure for a long time after therapy has been completed.

Radiation may also cause hair loss to the specific body part being treated. Although this is generally temporary, higher doses can also cause permanency. Unlike chemotherapy, radiation treatment does not cause generalized hair loss.

Fatigue, or generalized weakness, is another common side effect of radiation therapy. It tends to increase gradually and is cumulative as radiation continues.

Fatigue, or generalized weakness, is another common side effect of radiation therapy. It tends to increase gradually and is cumulative as radiation continues. After completion of a course of radiation therapy, many patients have a significant degree of fatigue.

Medical problems—including infection, anemia, and dehydration, all of which are treatable—can compound fatigue that is caused by radiation. Your physician should look for any of these aggravating factors. Ways of coping with fatigue include ensuring adequate sleep at night, resting during the day, eating a balanced diet with adequate calories and protein, and exercising at a tolerable level. Light exercise, such as walking and stretching, is helpful. A consultation with a physical therapist may prove helpful for advice on incorporating light exercise into your daily routine.

Radiation can cause a loss of appetite (anorexia) or nausea (Questions 66 and 68 on pages 147 and 150). Radiation treatments to the neck or chest may result in a sore throat or dry mouth, resulting in a condition called **xerostomia**, which results from damage to the salivary glands. Saliva is essential for chewing and swallowing food and is the primary lubricant for food. Inflammation

Xerostomia

Dryness of the mouth due to disease.

to the **esophagus** may also occur. This condition, called **esophagitis**, results in painful or difficult swallowing and possibly also heartburn.

If you experience esophagitis or xerostomia, consider eating softer foods or commercially available dietary shakes. You should avoid citrus fruits and juices, as these can be especially irritating. Commercially available saliva substitutes may also be helpful for coping with a dry mouth; your healthcare team can help with this.

Esophagus

The tube connecting the throat to the stomach.

Esophagitis

Inflammation of the esophagus.

CHEMOTHERAPY AND RADIATION THERAPY

PART FIVE

Other Therapies

What is immunotherapy?

What are monoclonal antibodies?

How are monoclonal antibodies administered?

More . . .

77. What is immunotherapy?

Immunotherapy, sometimes referred to as **biologic therapy**, is a treatment that involves the use of the immune system to treat the disease. These treatments include monoclonal antibodies and radioimmunotherapies, as well as allogeneic stem cell transplants.

One area of research has been the use of therapeutic vaccines to treat lymphoma or prevent its reoccurrence. A vaccine is usually a preparation of a protein given to stimulate an immune response to protect against particular infections. In lymphoma, vaccination has been experimental and used a protein obtained from lymphoma cells **idiotype** and was not present on normal cells. Unfortunately clinical trials were performed and did not demonstrate that this approach was effective.

78. What are monoclonal antibodies?

Monoclonal antibodies are immunoglobulin proteins that are produced by one population of cells or clone (hence monoclonal). Every antibody is built in the shape of the letter "Y." This structure allows the antibody to be useful for fighting infection. It also makes it useful for treating some types of cancer. The arms of the "Y" have a particular protein sequence that can recognize and attach to small, specific protein targets, termed "antigens." The foot of the "Y" can link to other cells in the immune system that can rid the body of the antigen. Antibodies are vital to a normal immune system, providing essential protection against otherwise potentially fatal infections.

Another way to help understand monoclonal antibodies is to know that we all have white blood cells that specialize

Biologic therapy

Treatment that focuses the body's immune system on diseased cells.

Idiotype

A protein sequence on the surface of B-lymphocytes that is like a fingerprint. All related lymphocytes contain the same protein sequence.

One area of research has been the use of therapeutic vaccines to treat lymphoma or prevent its reoccurrence.

in making antibodies. These plasma cells are the most mature B-cells in our immune system. Each plasma cell is responsible for one antibody. In turn, each antibody acts specifically against one specific antigen. Antigens are proteins located on the surface of all cells, which our immune system uses to determine whether cells are a necessary part of the body or need to be destroyed. Lymphoma treatments now available consist of large amounts of antibodies that can be specifically directed to a single antigen on a lymphoma cell's surface. An analogy often used is that the monoclonal antibody is a guided missile that hones in on lymphoma cells and destroys them.

CD20 is an antigen that is present on the lymphoma cells of most patients who have B-cell lymphomas. Rituximab (the first immunotherapy that the FDA approved for use in cancer) is an antibody that is designed so that the arms of the "Y" attach to CD20. When it is infused into the circulation, it seeks out the CD20 that is present on the lymphocytes and targets them for destruction. Since monoclonal antibodies only target the B cells involved in non-Hodgkin lymphoma and cause the immune system to destroy only those cells, it does not cause many of the side effects that normally come with chemotherapy or radiation treatment. Patients generally do not lose their hair or experience delayed nausea or vomiting and should be able to continue normal activities, including work.

Radioimmunotherapeutic antibodies are also approved for the treatment of indolent lymphoma. They also target CD20 but carry a payload in the form of a radioactive molecule. In this way, radiation is specifically delivered to the lymphoma cells, resulting in less damage to normal body cells. Other monoclonal antibodies are now available for patients with breast cancer and colon cancer, and many more are in clinical trials.

79. How are monoclonal antibodies administered?

Monoclonal antibodies are infused intravenously in varying schedules. For example, rituximab is commonly infused every week for 4 weeks in an outpatient setting. When rituximab is given along with chemotherapy, the schedule depends on the chemotherapy regimen. The side effects of this medication generally occur only while it is being administered. Overall, this treatment is very well tolerated with few long-term sequelae.

The first time rituximab is infused, patients are likely to experience fever and chills, which can be quite uncomfortable, but this resolves by slowing the infusion. These symptoms generally decrease with subsequent infusions.

Because of this, the first infusion takes the longest, maybe even more than 8 hours. Subsequent infusions can generally be completed in 90 minutes. Fever and chills occur less often with the remaining infusions. Acetaminophen (Tylenol®) and diphenhydramine (Benadryl®) given before the infusion (i.e., as premedications) can help to reduce the severity of the fever and chills. Brentuximab vedotin is administered intravenously every three weeks. Generally premedications are only used with brentuximab if patients have a reaction with the first infusion.

^{131}I tositumomab (Bexxar) and ^{90}Y ibritumomab tiuxetan (Zevalin) are more complicated to administer than unlabeled monoclonal antibodies such as rituximab. Because they are a form of radiation treatment (iodine or yttrium), a **nuclear medicine** physician or a radiation oncologist is required for their administration. Only one course of treatment is necessary, but it takes 7 to 14 days.

Nuclear medicine

The medicine specialty that deals with using radioisotopes for obtaining body scans and for treatment.

For ^{90}Y Ibritumomab tiuxetan, the monoclonal antibody rituximab is administered on the first day of treatment. Because of the need for special handling of radiation treatments, it may be necessary to receive the two treatments in different locations, which can be inconvenient. On days 7 to 9 of treatment, a second dose of rituximab is given. This is followed by the actual treatment dose of ^{90}Y ibritumomab tiuxetan, which only takes 10 minutes to infuse. The production of ^{131}I-tositumomab was discontinued in 2014.

A bone marrow examination is recommended before the administration of radiolabeled antibody therapy. If more than 25% of the marrow space is involved with lymphoma, these agents should not be given, as there is a risk that too much radiation will be concentrated in the marrow, possibly resulting in permanent or very long-lasting marrow damage. Blood counts will drop and they should be evaluated weekly for about 12 weeks.

80. What are targeted or molecular therapies?

Although monoclonal antibodies are functionally targeted therapies, this term is often used to refer to agents that act in a very focused and specific way inside cancer cells. As the biology of the abnormalities within cancer cells becomes better understood, scientists have begun to develop agents that take advantage of specific molecular differences or pathways within the cancer cells specifically. Examples of classes of presently approved therapies are bortezomib (a proteasome inhibitor), vorinostat (a histone deacetylase or HDAC inhibitor), and ibrutinib (a Bruton's tyrosine kinase inhibitor).

Proteasomes regulate the levels of certain proteins in normal cells. Cells need to continuously clear out proteins as part of normal function. Proteasomes are often referred to as the "garbage can" of the cell. They remove proteins that are no longer needed or functional and allow the cell to stay healthy. As cancer cells are so active in growth and division they make a lot of proteins. When the garbage can function is impaired (inhibited) in a cancer cell by a proteasome inhibitor, the trash (certain proteins) builds up and this appears to impair continued cancer cell growth. Bortezomib is a proteasome inhibitor approved for use in myeloma and relapsed mantle cell lymphoma. It was developed for use by intravenous injection. A very common side effect of bortezomib is peripheral neuropathy (numbness and tingling or pain in the fingers and toes; constipation). Giving the medicine less often and/or by subcutaneous rather than intravenous injection appears to lessen the degree of neuropathy.

Histones are proteins that help regulate how tightly or loosely "wrapped" the DNA inside cells is. Histone deacetylases induce histones to wrap the DNA more tightly, limiting the expression of certain genes. HDAC inhibitors interfere with the function of histone deacetylases, leading to more "loosely wound" DNA in certain regions. When the DNA is more loosely wound certain genes will be expressed to a greater degree. If the particular genes expressed make proteins that limit cell growth and division, this would limit cell growth. Vorinostat (taken by mouth) and romadepsin (taken by intravenous injection) are HDAC inhibitors approved for use in T-cell lymphomas. Both are approved for patients with cutaneous T-cell lymphomas who have received prior systemic therapy. Romadepsin is also approved for patients with peripheral T-cell lymphomas who have received at least one prior therapy. Common side effects include nausea, diminished appetite, diarrhea, and low platelet counts.

Bruton's tyronsine kinase is an enzyme that is part of a critical signaling process inside the cell. This enzyme affects the generation of proteins that induce cell growth and division. Inhibiting this enzyme appears to limit the generation of those proteins, thereby limiting the growth of the cells. Ibrutinib is a recently approved specific inhibitor of this enzyme. It is taken by mouth and is approved for patients with CLL or mantle cell lymphoma who have received at least one prior therapy. Common side effects include low blood counts, fatigue and diarrhea. There appears to be a small risk of bleeding with this agent for reasons that are not presently well understood, so reporting any unusual bruising or bleeding to your physician would be very important.

81. What is a bone marrow or stem cell transplant?

A bone marrow or stem cell transplant is a treatment that either allows for the administration of higher doses of chemotherapy or radiation than you could receive without the transplant (autologous stem cell transplants), or takes advantage of the ability to place a new set of stem cells/immune system into a patient (allogeneic stem cell transplant), or some element of both. The effects of most chemotherapy drugs on the patient's bone marrow limit the ability to significantly increase the dose of many drugs that are used to treat lymphoma. Being able to increase the dose of the drugs can reduce the chance that the lymphoma will return. In the case of some chemotherapy drugs, this increased dose could destroy the bone marrow or suppress it for very long periods of time. In this situation, the prolonged period of low white cell counts and low platelets would substantially increase the risk of infection and bleeding respectively. During the period of low blood counts, patients generally require regular transfusions of red blood cells and platelets as well as antibiotics and white cell growth factors such as G-CSF (Neupogen®) to support the marrow in the best way possible until the counts returned. In order to shorten the period of low blood counts (or to replace the existing marrow/immune system, or both) a bone marrow or stem cell transplant can be performed.

A bone marrow transplant, as the name suggests, involves actually using the bone marrow stem cells for the transplant. Obtaining the bone marrow requires an operation with a general anesthetic. This procedure is performed less commonly now, and most transplant centers obtain stem cells from the peripheral circulation rather than directly from the bone marrow. Such transplants are called peripheral blood stem cell transplants. Although obtained from the blood, the stem cells are still bone marrow stem cells, but they move into the bloodstream after treatment with growth factors such as G-CSF (Neupogen®). Stem cells also move into the blood circulation as blood counts recover after chemotherapy. Often a patient's own stem cells are collected after the administration of both chemotherapy and white blood cell growth factors. When transplanted back into the patient after the high-dose chemotherapy regimen has been completed, the stem cells are able to produce red cells, white cells, and platelets, decreasing the duration of time that the blood counts remain low, and decreasing the chances of complications resulting from the low counts. Using stem cells obtained from the blood results in a significantly shorter period of low blood counts compared to the use of bone marrow. This has enabled patients to have shorter hospital stays or possibly even to have such a treatment performed as an outpatient.

82. Why is a transplant used for treating lymphoma?

Basically, there are two main mechanisms by which a transplant can be useful in treating lymphoma. First as described previously, it enables the safer delivery of much higher doses of chemotherapy than would otherwise be possible without the availability of such cells. The higher doses of chemotherapy may cure an aggressive lymphoma not curable with lower doses of chemotherapy, or prevent an indolent lymphoma from returning for a longer period of time than after regular doses of chemotherapy. An **allogeneic transplant** (i.e., using somebody else's bone marrow or peripheral blood cells) offers the additional advantage of providing normal stem cells from a healthy donor. Therefore, there is no chance of lymphoma cells being returned with the transplant. Also, any damaged stem cells from previous chemotherapy or radiation used to treat lymphoma are replaced by new normal and healthy marrow cells. The risk of secondary malignancies including myelodysplasia and leukemia should be eliminated. However the main reason for performing an allogeneic transplant is the introduction of the donor's immune system into the patient. In some types of lymphoma, the donors' immune system can then recognize lymphoma cells remaining in the patient, see them as foreign, and destroy them. In this way, an allogeneic transplant is a potential cure for some types of lymphoma. This effect is called the **graft-versus-lymphoma (GVL)** effect (see Question 90 on page 187). Unfortunately, similar types of immune cells from the healthy donor that cause GVL

OTHER THERAPIES

Allogeneic transplant

A transplant using another individual as the donor.

Graft-versus-lymphoma (GVL)

A situation in which the donor's immune system recognizes the recipient's lymphoma cells as foreign and works to eliminate the lymphoma.

can cause GVHD in the patient as well (see Question 88 on page 184). In this condition, the donor's immune cells recognize the patient's tissues and organs as foreign, attacking them immunologically. GVHD can often be treated and controlled but sometimes can cause a more serious problem or even death. The chance that GVHD will occur and perhaps be more difficult to control rises significantly for older patients with donors who are less well tissue-type matched to the patient. A randomized controlled study evaluated autologous and allogeneic bone marrow transplants to determine the better approach to treating indolent lymphoma. This study was not completed as patients were reluctant to be enrolled. Data to help answer this question was obtained from registry data. Allogeneic transplants were resulting in longer remissions with decreased relapses than occurred following autologous transplants but the allogeneic transplants were associated with a higher risk of death and this offset any advantage seen with an allogeneic transplant. This and other transplant-related problems are reasons why an allogeneic transplant is not often considered a good choice for older patients, or early in the course of a lymphoma when simpler therapies offer much less risk with good treatment results. GVHD and GVL occur only with an allogeneic transplant. An autologous transplant does not have the benefit of GVL. It therefore relies on the high doses of chemotherapy to cure or treat the lymphoma. Because of the immune benefit of GVL, allogeneic transplants do not necessarily need high doses of chemotherapy. It has now been fairly clearly demonstrated that delivering much smaller doses of chemotherapy to patients before the allogeneic cells are infused can be associated with very good results. In these circumstances, large doses of chemotherapy may not be required (e.g., for a patient in remission already) or desirable for safety reasons (e.g., for an older patient or a patient who previously had an autologous stem cell transplant). In these cases, the transplant relies much more on the GVL effect. These types of transplants are often referred to as **nonmyeloablative or reduced intensity allogeneic stem cell transplants**. This has allowed allogeneic stem cell transplants and the GVL effect to be extended to patients in whom previously it would have been too unsafe, and has demonstrated a decrease in the risk of complications that may arise from more intense pre-transplant chemotherapy regimens. (**Table 15** and Question 89 on page 186).

83. What is an autologous transplant?

An autologous transplant uses your own bone marrow or blood stem cells to restore the blood counts after high-dose chemotherapy. It is used to treat many types of lymphoma, including Hodgkin lymphoma and many subtypes of non-Hodgkin lymphoma. The circumstance when an autologous transplant is helpful is one in which the lymphoma is likely to respond to much higher doses of chemotherapy than can be given without

Nonmyeloablative or reduced intensity allogeneic stem cell transplants

A transplant in which the doses of chemotherapy or radiotherapy are reduced compared to those given for a standard transplant.

OTHER THERAPIES

Table 15 Different Types of Bone Marrow or Blood Stem Cell Transplants

Transplant type	Source of stem cells	Preparative regimen
Autologous	Stem cells obtained from the patient's own blood or bone marrow	High-dose therapy
Allogeneic	Matched stem cells from a	High-dose therapy
Sibling	Sibling	
Unrelated donor	Volunteer donor	
Cord blood transplant	Unbilical cord blood stem cell bank	
Reduced intensity (nonmyeloablative)	Sibling or unrelated donor	Reduced-dose therapy

the transplant. The higher doses of chemotherapy can also destroy the bone marrow. Therefore, before giving the high-dose therapy, stem cells are collected from the patient and are frozen. After the high-dose chemotherapy, the stem cells are thawed and infused back into the patient through a central venous catheter. The stem cells rapidly find their way back to the marrow, and after a period of usually 10–14 days post infusion, the stem cells start making all of the different types of blood cells. The cells that recover most rapidly are the white blood cells. The number of stem cells obtained before the transplant affects to some extent how fast the blood cells, particularly platelets, recover. Faster recovery generally occurs with higher numbers of stem cells. For appropriate patients, the risks of an autologous transplant are low. Because the blood counts drop after the high-dose chemotherapy, there is a higher risk of infection. If this occurs, intravenous antibiotics are required. Platelet transfusions are often needed to reduce the risk of bleeding, and blood transfusions are often required to manage anemia.

Many transplant centers perform autologous transplants on an outpatient basis. When you receive it as an outpatient, it is important that you have someone available at home to help and to drive you to the hospital for the frequent visits (often daily) that are required. If any complication such as a fever occurs, you would be admitted to the hospital.

84. How is an autologous transplant performed?

The procedure for an autologous transplant involves a number of steps. If your lymphoma specialist recommends an autologous transplant, a number of tests are necessary to try to ensure that you are well enough to tolerate the high-dose therapy and the following period of low blood counts. These tests include evaluations of your heart, lung, and kidney function in addition to an assessment of your general well-being. Blood tests to detect any infections, such as hepatitis, will also be obtained. Approval from your insurance company is also required. Next, an **apheresis catheter**, which is usually placed in the upper chest wall, is necessary for collecting stem cells from your blood. **Stem cell mobilization** is the next step, whereby the bone marrow stem cells are stimulated to move into the blood circulation. For stem cell mobilization, white blood cell growth factors given alone or sometimes after further chemotherapy have been administered. The stem cell collection will then be scheduled as the white blood cell count recovers. The collection of the stem cells involves a procedure called **leukapheresis**, for which you are connected to a leukapheresis machine via your apheresis catheter. A small amount of your blood volume is transferred into the machine where the white blood cells are separated from the red blood cells and the platelets. The white cells contain the bone marrow stem cells and are collected in a special bag to be frozen. The red cells and platelets are returned to your circulation. The leukapheresis often needs to be repeated over a few days in order to get an adequate number of stem cells. The procedure on the machine takes approximately 4 to 6 hours. For patients who have difficulty mobilizing enough cells, often because of prior chemotherapy, a medication known as plerixafor may be added to the growth factor medication to improve mobilization and collection.

The stem cells are then frozen along with a chemical protectant called dimethyl sulfoxide (DMSO), which

Apheresis catheter

A large indwelling catheter placed through the skin into a large vein to allow the collection of stem cells.

Stem cell mobilization

The process by which bone marrow stem cells are stimulated to move into blood circulation.

Leukapheresis

A procedure to remove large numbers of white blood cells from the body.

OTHER THERAPIES

is responsible for the strange garlic-like taste and smell that patients and families usually notice when the stem cells are infused back into the patient. The next stage of the transplant involves managing the side effects of the high-dose chemotherapy and awaiting the recovery of the blood counts. The transplant team will discuss common side effects of the high-dose chemotherapy with you.

85. What are the complications of an autologous transplant?

Problems can relate to having an apheresis catheter, the leukapheresis procedure, the high doses of chemo-therapy, and the resulting low blood counts before bone marrow recovery.

The overall risk and rate of life-threatening complications from an autologous transplant for patients in otherwise good health are very low and minimal.

The overall risk and rate of life-threatening complica-tions from an autologous transplant for patients in oth-erwise good health are very low and minimal. The first problem to present itself could be as a result of the apher-esis catheter. These complications are similar to those that can occur with the placement of a central venous catheter, as discussed in Question 62 on page 144.

Peripheral blood stem cells are collected via a process called apheresis or leukapheresis. This procedure is gen-erally painless. The leukapheresis machine removes a small amount of your blood volume at a time, separating the bone marrow stem cells from the other blood cells. Patients are closely monitored to ensure that too much blood is not removed at any one time. Sometimes diz-ziness (lightheadedness or a feeling of faintness) may occur. If so, the machine settings can be adjusted, or a little extra fluid can be given to adjust for the blood volume that is outside of the body at any time. In addition, because the blood outside of the body cannot be allowed to clot, an anticoagulant is added to your blood that can bind calcium. This can result in a fall in the blood calcium that may result in tingling in the fingers and face. Again, adjustments can be made to the machine settings to compensate for these abnormalities, or you may be given extra calcium (such as calcium carbonate [e.g., Tums®]). Therefore, it is important to inform your nurse if you are experiencing any discomfort. If you have a low platelet count before leukapheresis, the procedure can result in a further fall, and you may need a platelet transfusion before the procedure.

The conditioning or preparative regimens, meaning the high-dose chemotherapy and/or radiation given the week prior to the transplant, vary according to the type of lymphoma being treated, the patient's overall condition, and the medical center in which the transplant is being performed. These treatments may cause nausea and vomiting, which can be reduced with good antinausea drugs; thus, severe nausea is much less common these days. Hair loss, although common, is specific to the combination of drugs used in the conditioning regimen. It usually starts a week or so following the chemotherapy. When this begins, you may prefer to shave your head, as the continuing hair loss can be quite messy. Chemotherapy can damage the lining of the gut. The mouth, all of the way through to the anus, can be affected, resulting in mouth pain, chest pain similar to heartburn, abdominal pain, diarrhea, and rectal pain. Different chemotherapy regimens cause this to varying degrees. Medication can keep you comfortable if the pain becomes unpleasant. A regimen of mouth care that is designed to maintain high levels of oral hygiene will be started with the high-dose chemotherapy. Frequent mouth cleaning with sponges and a mouthwash will lessen the chance of complications, although it may not prevent breakdown. The high doses of chemotherapy can occasionally have damaging effects on other normal body parts. The degree to which this happens depends on the exact type of drug used, and your transplant team will discuss this with you. Possible but uncommon side effects include damage to the lungs, heart, liver, bladder, or kidneys. During the time that chemotherapy is given and in the days afterward, you will be examined daily to assess for any evidence of organ damage from the chemotherapy. Blood tests are also obtained for the same reason. Rare complications can arise even after you appear to have completely recovered from the transplant and have returned home. One such side effect relates to the very active drug carmustine that can be used for treating lymphoma and is commonly used in the high-dose therapy regimens. It can cause an inflammation in the lungs, referred to as **BCNU pneumonitis**, which can result in a cough, shortness of breath, or a fever developing even up to a year after the transplant. It can be effectively treated with a course of steroids. Therefore, if these symptoms develop, you should contact your physician without delay.

BCNU pneumonitis

Inflammation of the lungs caused by the chemotherapy drug BCNU.

GVHD does not occur after an autologous transplant. Immune-suppressing medications are therefore not required. Patients do not normally need to be on steroids after an autologous transplantation.

Low blood counts are an expected temporary side effect of an autologous transplant, and problems related to it are discussed in Questions 69 and 70 on pages 151 and 153.

86. What is an allogeneic transplant?

An allogeneic transplant uses stem cells from a donor. The source of these stem cells can be bone marrow, peripheral blood, or umbilical cord blood. Stem cells are special cells that can produce all three blood cell components. These are white blood cells, red blood cells, and platelets. The donor generally needs to be compatible in terms of genetic similarities. To ensure this, special testing referred to as **human leukocyte antigen (HLA) typing** is performed on both the patient and potential donors.

The HLA system consists of a set of different proteins present on most cells in the body. Eight of these proteins are very important for the purposes of a transplant and are transmitted from your parents in two groups of four proteins each. The four proteins in each group are usually passed on together. Each parent provides one set of the proteins to each child. As one of the sets comes from each parent, there is a 25% chance that each brother and sister, as long as they share the same parents, will have the same set of proteins and therefore will have identical HLA. It is rare for other relatives besides brothers or sisters to be HLA identical, as they do not share parents and, therefore, have inherited different HLA proteins. In rare situations, however, it is worthwhile to test children or parents. A stem cell transplant performed with stem cells obtained from an identical twin is called a syngeneic transplant.

If there are no matched siblings, an allogeneic transplant may still be possible, but an unrelated donor would then need to be found. A transplant using an HLA-identical donor other than a sibling is referred to as a

Human leukocyte antigen (HLA) typing

Testing of the transplantation antigens to determine whether two people are compatible for transplantation.

matched unrelated donor transplant. An organization, the National Marrow Donor Program, maintains a registry of millions of partly to completely HLA-typed volunteers who are prepared to donate marrow or peripheral blood stem cells. For HLA typing, a blood sample is obtained, and a bone marrow evaluation is unnecessary. If you are a possible candidate for an unrelated donor transplant, you can be referred to a transplant center, where a search of the registry can be initiated.

The side effects and risks of an allogeneic transplant are quite different from those of an autologous transplant. The fundamental reason is that, along with the new bone marrow cells, you acquire the immune system of your donor. This can be beneficial due to the GVL effect whereby the new immune cells recognize lymphoma cells as foreign and act to eliminate them. This can result in treatment benefits that are unavailable using only chemotherapy. The downside is GVHD (discussed in Question 89 on page 186).

87. How is an allogeneic transplant performed?

An allogeneic transplant differs from an autologous transplant in a number of ways. Two people are involved—you and your donor. For matched unrelated donor transplants, the National Marrow Donor Program arranges the collection or harvesting of the donor stem cells. These are obtained either directly from the bone marrow during a surgical procedure with general anesthesia or from the blood circulation using leukapheresis. If leukapheresis is performed, as discussed in Question 85 on page 178, the donor receives a white blood cell growth factor to stimulate stem cells into the blood. Once the stem cells are obtained, they are shipped to the transplant center for infusion into the patient. Before stem cell collection, a physician evaluates and screens the donor for any illness or infectious disease that would make it unsafe. In cases in which the donor is a family member, your transplant physician will arrange for stem cell collection. Once obtained, the stem cells can be either frozen or infused directly into the transplant recipient. Whether they are fresh or frozen, there is no difference in outcome to the recipient. The therapy given just before you receive the transplant is designed, except in the case of a nonmyeloablative transplant, to try to eliminate any remaining lymphoma. It is also designed to eliminate your bone marrow and immune system to ensure that your immune system does not reject the new bone marrow cells. The high-dose therapy may consist of chemotherapy alone or may be combined with radiation therapy to the whole body (called total body irradiation). You will generally be hospitalized for these treatments, although in some centers, the radiation may be arranged as an outpatient treatment, usually twice a day over 3 days.

Medications will be provided to prevent nausea and vomiting. After the chemotherapy, a rest day is usual to allow for elimination of drugs from the body. The new bone marrow stem cells are then infused into your bloodstream through a catheter. The day that you receive the new stem cells is referred to as day 0. Then the waiting period for the new cells to start producing all of the blood cells begins. During this period, your blood counts will be low, and the risks for an infection are highest. You will likely also need platelet and red cell transfusions. The chemotherapy or total body irradiation often results in **mucositis**, which can last for a number of days. Morphine may be required for adequate pain control.

Mucositis

Inflamation of any of the mucous membranes lining the digestive tract from the mouth, down to the esophogus, to the anus.

Your transplant team will observe you closely to guard against and manage any complications that may arise. After a period of 10 to 14 days, but sometimes as long as 3 weeks, the new stem cells begin to produce blood cells. The white blood count is usually the first of the blood types to recover, often rising to a normal level over a period of only a few days. It is during the time of white cell recovery and the following weeks that GVHD is most likely to occur. The platelet count recovers more slowly than the white count.

88. What is GVHD?

GVHD is the syndrome in which lymphocytes derived from the donor graft can recognize the recipient's body as foreign. The donor lymphocytes essentially attempt to reject the recipient's body. In a kidney or liver transplant patient with a normal immune system, antirejection drugs are given to prevent the patient from rejecting the new kidney or liver. In the case of a bone marrow recipient, his or her immune system has been eliminated, and thus, the new transplanted immune system attempts to reject the recipient. GVHD can be either acute or chronic. Acute GVHD tends to occur when white cells first appear or in the weeks after the transplant. Characteristically, it affects the skin, liver, and/or the gut. It can cause a rash that can affect any area, but in milder cases it may affect only the palms and soles as well as the ear lobes. When the gut is affected, diarrhea occurs. Blood tests or the presence of jaundice can indicate liver involvement.

There are several medications given to prevent GVHD— cyclosporine, tacrolimus, sirolimus, and mycophenolate mofetil are the most commonly used. Another drug called methotrexate, a chemotherapy drug, is also useful in low doses after the transplant to prevent GVHD. You may be given one or a combination of two or three. In certain circumstances for an unrelated donor transplant, a medication called antithymocyte globulin may also be given both to promote engraftment and to reduce the incidence of severe GVHD.

Acute GVHD is scored from 1 to 4 according to the severity of the rash, diarrhea, and the abnormal liver tests. If it is grade 1, your transplant physician may choose not to treat it, because some degree of GVHD can be beneficial, as **GVL** may accompany the GVHD. In cases in which the GVHD is more severe, treatment is needed.

GVL
Graft-versus-lymphoma

The first treatment for GVHD is usually a steroid, which is given orally or intravenously. The medicines used in the attempt to prevent GVHD are also continued. Other medications will be added if the steroids fail to control the GVHD. However acute GVHD that does not respond to steroids is an extremely difficult situation to rectify.

Chronic GVHD may occur at any time after the transplant. It may follow directly from acute GVHD or arise without the occurrence of acute GVHD. Chronic GVHD affects individuals differently than does acute GVHD. It may result in dry eyes or a dry mouth. It can affect the skin, resulting in skin thickening. If severe, this can affect the joints, resulting in stiffening. The treatment of chronic GVHD is similar to acute GVHD, but there is increasing evidence that medications such as thalidomide and imatinib can be beneficial.

89. What are reduced intensity conditioning (RIC) and nonmyloablative allogeneic stem cell transplants?

These types of transplant are modifications of the original concept of an allogeneic stem cell transplant. With these transplants, the intensity of the chemotherapy/radiation therapy given prior to the transplant is reduced modestly (RIC) or substantially (nonmyeloablative). RIC and nonmyeloablative transplants rely more on the effects of GVL to produce the treatment effect. Reasons to utilize these types of transplants are many. In some circumstances, the lymphoma may already be in a very good state of remission, and there may not be a reason to require large doses of chemotherapy or radiotherapy prior to the transplant. In other cases, the lymphoma may be slow growing but also very resistant to chemotherapy such that the addition of even large doses of chemotherapy/radiotherapy may not be expected to shrink the tumor further. In this situation, large doses of chemotherapy may simply add side effects and risks to the treatment without any significant likelihood of improving the outcomes. Finally, in older or sicker patients who may not tolerate larger doses of chemotherapy, the ability to use smaller doses allows the benefits of GVL to be offered to a broader spectrum and age range of patients. In this type of transplant, the lower dose of chemotherapy or radiation given before receiving the donor stem cells is also intended to prevent rejection of the new cells (by suppressing the patient's immune system prior to the transplant), not so much to eliminate residual lymphoma. The idea is that the new immune system will work to eliminate the lymphoma. This takes time, and therefore this type of transplant is generally not felt to be suitable for patients with rapidly growing lymphoma.

Also, the best GVL effect is seen among patients with indolent lymphomas since their growth rate is slower, allowing the GVL effect to take hold before the tumor can substantially progress. It appears likely that the complication rate for this sort of transplant is lower, partly because it has less effect on normal body tissues from the lower doses of chemotherapy. Tissue damage contributes to GVHD by releasing cytokines. In the RIC transplant setting, this is minimized with—it is hoped—less GVHD while still allowing GVL to occur. One major research goal in transplant is to separate the cells causing GVHD from those that can cause GVL. Currently, this goal remains elusive.

90. What is GVL?

When an allogeneic stem cell transplant is performed, the newly transplanted donor immune system will generally perceive the patient's (i.e., host's) body and tissues as foreign. The immune reaction against the normal host tissues is known as GVHD (see Question 88 on page 184). However the newly transplanted immune system can also potentially recognize residual lymphoma cells in the patient as foreign as well. The stem cell graft's immunological attack directed against malignant cells is obviously potentially beneficial as it can kill lymphoma cells that were not killed by any prior chemotherapy. This is known as the GVL effect. It is an important strategic difference between an autologous and an allogeneic transplant. The observation that relapses are less common after allogeneic transplants compared to autologous transplants is likely based largely on this GVL effect. If a patient relapses after an allogeneic transplant, it is sometimes possible to attain another remission after the infusion of donor lymphocytes alone if the original donor is available to donate such cells. The observation that less intense (e.g., RIC) transplant regimens can be very effective in indolent lymphomas is an illustration of the potency of the GVL effect in certain situations.

91. When should I have a transplant?

This is a complicated issue and depends on your type of lymphoma, your response to previous treatment, your age, and your overall general condition. The answer is therefore addressed depending on lymphoma type.

Indolent Lymphoma

Because indolent lymphoma tends to occur in older individuals, most patients are not candidates for a full dose or traditional allogeneic transplant. A RIC or non-myeloablative transplant can be considered in certain circumstances. Some studies suggest that this type of transplant may actually cure some patients through the benefits of the GVL effect (see Question 90 on page 187). This treatment option should be considered, especially in younger patients with a suitable donor. However, because of the risks inherent with this type of transplant, it is often offered after 2 or more prior therapies (possibly including an autologous transplant) have been tried and failed. It should be considered before the lymphoma is resistant to usual therapies because this type of transplant generally works best when patients are in a reasonable state of remission prior to the transplant being performed.

An autologous transplant is an option for a greater number of patients. Most lymphoma physicians feel that it does not provide a cure for many, or perhaps any patients, but in many instances it can provide an extended period of remission before the lymphoma returns. Because autologous transplants have a low risk of serious complications, they are frequently considered. Extending the time before another course of treatment is needed may be a significant advantage for many patients. Some studies suggest that survival may be slightly prolonged by the use of autologous stem cell transplants in the setting of relapsed indolent lymphomas.

Many clinical studies are being conducted in an attempt to improve the results of autologous transplants. Such studies include attempts to purge the bone marrow stem cells before the transplant. **Purging** refers to the removal of any lymphoma cells that may contaminate the stem cells. Currently, methods of purging include treating the patient with chemotherapy or antibodies before collecting the stem cells. It is not yet clear whether this attempt to reduce or eliminate the presence of lymphoma cells in the graft (i.e., purging) results in a better outcome. Ongoing studies are addressing the ability of maintenance therapy to prevent lymphoma recurrence after an autologous transplant. Such approaches include the use of monoclonal antibody treatments.

Purging

The technique whereby certain cells (usually cancerous) are removed from the remaining cells present in the collected bone marrow or stem cells.

Aggressive Lymphoma

The GVL effect that can cure some indolent lymphomas in general appears to be less effective for aggressive lymphomas. Therefore, an allogeneic transplant is performed less frequently for these disorders with the exception perhaps of some of the T-cell lymphomas. However, for many patients whose lymphoma returns after the initial CHOP (with or without monoclonal antibodies), an autologous transplant is often the next recommended treatment (see Question 84 on page 177). Remember, these lymphomas can still be cured with a transplant. As previously noted, patients whose lymphoma continues to respond to regular doses of chemotherapy are the best candidates for transplantation. There may also be patients who, at the time their lymphoma is first diagnosed, appear to be at a particularly high risk of the lymphoma recurring after chemotherapy. The IPI can help to identify such patients. At the present time, the benefits of autologous transplants in first remission for patients with aggressive lymphomas remain unclear (particularly in the rituximab and PET era) and there does not appear to be a group of patients in whom this should routinely be considered.

Hodgkin Lymphoma

Hodgkin lymphoma is curable in a significant number of patients with radiation therapy, chemotherapy, or a combination of both.

Hodgkin lymphoma is curable in a significant number of patients with radiation therapy, chemotherapy, or a combination of both. If the lymphoma recurs after you have received only radiation, chemotherapy alone may cure the disease. If the recurrence follows chemotherapy, especially if it returns within a short period after completing the therapy, a transplant may be necessary. Most often, an autologous transplant is recommended, but in some situations an allogeneic transplant will be recommended.

92. Should I seek complementary therapy?

Conventional therapies, including such treatments as chemotherapy, monoclonal antibody therapy, and radiation therapy, are treatments that medical doctors recommend. These treatments have been demonstrated in clinical trials to provide the most anticancer activity. Obviously, these treatments are far from perfect, and much work remains to be done. Because of the failings of conventional treatments, interest in **complementary therapy** and alternative therapy is high.

Complementary therapies are techniques or approaches that are used in addition to standard or conventional treatments. Examples include meditation, acupuncture, relaxation and massage, visualization, and diet and herbal regimens. Many of these treatments are derived from traditional healing practices and can be important additions to the more traditional treatments. They often help individuals to cope better and feel more in control. Oncologists recognize many complementary therapies for their positive effects on a patient's sense of well-being. The medical community accepts and encourages therapies such as relaxation and visualization. In many cancer centers, you can receive instruction and learn the techniques of various complementary therapies. It is advisable to discuss these therapies with your physician. Rarely, there may be specific reasons why you should avoid a specific complementary therapy.

Meditation and relaxation have been demonstrated to help obtain relief from nausea, anxiety, depression, and stress. Many ways exist to practice meditation and relaxation, and many books and tapes are available at libraries and bookstores. You may need to experiment with a few different techniques before you find one that works for you.

The positive effects of such complementary techniques on the outcome of lymphoma are unknown. Although there is no concrete evidence that such techniques can directly influence lymphoma, indirect effects may exist via subtle changes in the immune system. No harm is brought from such interventions, especially if they help patients to feel more in control. Additional information can be obtained from the National Center for Complementary and Alternative Medicine. Its Web site is at www.nccam.nih.gov.

93. Should I seek alternative therapy?

Alternative therapy

A therapy other than a conventionally accepted medical treatment.

Alternative therapy, in contrast to complementary therapy, is the substitution of standard medical treatments with unproven and unconventional treatments. In many cases, even lymphoma that has recurred may be curable, so it is heartbreaking to see vulnerable patients decline such potentially curable therapy for alternative remedies without proven benefit. The use of such therapies may result in the loss of an opportunity for a cure.

Lymphoma patients, like all cancer patients, are vulnerable and may be disillusioned with their physician or medical clinic or feel bitter as a result of a relapse. In these situations, it is natural to reach out toward any hope.

Many claims are made for many different remedies. Often, the actual nature of the remedy is not disclosed, and such treatments may cost large sums of money. Usually, little or no evidence supports the use of the remedy apart from a list of testimonials from cured patients.

We would simply advise caution. You expect your lymphoma specialist to have a good rationale for the treatments that he or she prescribes. Hold alternative therapy practitioners to the same standard. Often, alternative therapy practitioners will state that only large pharmaceutical companies can afford to conduct such research. It has been suggested that these same companies even obstruct alternative therapy practitioners from conducting such research. Whatever the reason for the lack of studies and evidence regarding these treatments, it is unconscionable to make such exaggerated claims about expensive products to vulnerable patients. Furthermore, patients are often led to believe that the failure of a product was due to their lack of effort or belief in the product, and that with only more effort or belief (and of course expense) benefit may arise.

It is important to remember that all therapies considered standard for cancer patients have proven their value in high quality clinical trials. It is not particularly difficult to be able to make claims based on good outcomes of trials with small numbers of patients, or patients who were in some way intentionally or even unintentionally picked to be the best of the best. Most investigators have even seen the results of some of their own trials look very promising or even better than other standard therapies of the time until such therapies were compared in larger, better-controlled (e.g., randomized) trials. There are countless examples in oncology of therapies that looked good in early small trials only to be shown to be inferior or no better in subsequent larger, better-designed trials. The other important thing to understand is that clinical trials that are published in high-quality journals have been rigorously reviewed by experts. These experts were not involved in the study to ensure the highest quality of unbiased review, reporting, and conclusions, and great care is taken not to let such studies over-state their results or benefits. Very little can be said in a scientific manner with respect to any type of therapy that lacks this level of data.

94. What are clinical trials?

Clinical trials are the mechanism by which new and safer treatments are evaluated. They aim to determine whether a treatment is effective, whether it is better than existing treatments, and whether the treatment can be administered safely. It is only through carefully performed clinical trials that potential new treatments can be transferred from the laboratory to the bedside.

In the development of a new drug, preclinical studies are the first step. These are studies performed in laboratories and/or animals (usually mice). These studies provide the first indication that the drug has some activity directed against a cancer, and some estimation of the expectable side effects at various doses. If a drug appears promising, a phase 1 study may be performed, which is primarily conducted to determine the correct dose of the new treatment and to obtain further information about side effects. Most phase 1 studies are designed to start off at a very low dose of the medication in small groups of patients. The patients are monitored closely for the development of any side effects. If no side effects are seen, another small group of patients will be treated at a higher dose. In this fashion, subsequent patients receive increasing doses of the drug, assuming that the patients treated at the lower dose levels tolerated the medication without unacceptable side effects. In this way, the effect of the drug in humans can be assessed in a relatively safe manner. Of course, there are risks to participating in a phase 1 trial. Although unexpected side effects may exist, the possibility of obtaining a significant benefit also has potential. Often, it is patients whose cancer is progressing in spite of nearly all known standard treatments who are the most appropriate subjects to participate in phase 1 clinical trials.

After completing phase 1, new treatments enter phase 2 studies. Once the correct dose and side effects are known, the phase 2 study is to establish that a treatment is effective. A phase 2 study involves a larger group of patients who all generally receive the same dose. They are evaluated to determine how the cancer responds to the treatment and also to gather further information about side effects.

If the treatment still appears promising, it will continue into phase 3, which is usually designed to compare the new treatment with other currently available treatments. This phase often involves a randomized study in which patients have a 1-in-2 chance of receiving the new treatment. Patients are then followed closely, and the response of patients in the two groups is compared. If possible, it is preferable that neither the patient nor his or her physician is aware of which treatment is administered, as this could lead to bias in favor of one treatment over another. A phase 3 study is the best method for demonstrating that one treatment is better than another. The FDA has a mandate to regulate medications. Before approval for use, all clinical trial data are reviewed to ensure that a drug meets the standards for being safe and effective.

Only through clinical trials can patients and their doctors know which treatments are best for their type of cancer. A new treatment gets evaluated because there are indications that it may be more effective, safer, or easier on the patient than an alternative treatment. Drugs that do not show promise are not further evaluated. If clinical trials were not conducted, physicians would have nothing concrete to guide them when making recommendations to patients. Treatments currently used for lymphoma are the direct result of previous patients volunteering for clinical trials. The dramatic improvements in survival seen among patients with Hodgkin lymphoma and children with leukemia are direct results of clinical trials that sequentially incorporated advances from earlier studies into subsequent studies to allow for a steady path of successive improvements in outcomes.

Patients entering a clinical trial are not guinea pigs. Before a clinical trial can enroll patients, it is carefully reviewed from scientific, safety, and ethical viewpoints. Patients also need to provide informed consent, which establishes that they understand the reason for the study, the risks and possible benefits, and the availability of alternative treatment options. **Institutional review boards (IRB)** are required to approve and monitor the conduct of clinical trials and have the ability to suspend or close a trial if there are concerns about safety.

Institutional review board (IRB)

A group that reviews research studies to ensure they are safe and ethical.

A drug company with an interest in developing a particular drug may sponsor a clinical trial, or the funding may come from an independent source such as a university grant or a government agency. The same strict requirements need to be followed regardless of the source of funding.

95. Should I enter a clinical trial?

Participation in a clinical trial can be beneficial in many respects. You may be eligible to participate in various trials depending on your type and grade of lymphoma. Your overall condition and the treatment you have already received are also factors to be considered. Discuss with your lymphoma doctor whether any suitable clinical trials are available, as they often offer a way for receiving new and innovative treatments that otherwise may be unavailable. Patients in a clinical trial also receive very close medical supervision and monitoring.

Clinical trials are necessary because they help expand the knowledge base of lymphoma and the best treatment options now and in the future. Participants of clinical trials may have the opportunity to benefit from treatments that have shown promise in earlier research.

Cancer centers often have a number of clinical trials available for different cancers. Smaller oncology practices, however, may have few or no trials available. Participation in a trial may then require travel away from home and loved ones. Because a clinical trial cannot offer any guarantee of benefit, the disruption and inconvenience may outweigh the benefit and can also be a significant emotional and financial burden for you and your family.

When deciding on participation in a clinical trial, collect as much information as possible. Find out what the treatment involves, how it is different from standard treatments, and what the relative risks and benefits are. Ask whether any other clinical trials are available and what the experience has been to date. Inquire whether the trial is phase 1, phase 2, or phase 3, and ask what question the trial is hoping to answer.

Before making a final decision, ensure that you have a very good understanding of the treatment involved and also of the time commitment. Find out whether there are any costs for which you are responsible. Also, try to develop an understanding of the likelihood of benefit from the treatment. Thoughtful discussion with your physician and sometimes a second opinion may help you to make a rational decision.

Participation in a clinical trial can be beneficial in many respects. You may be eligible to participate in various trials depending on your type and grade of lymphoma.

OTHER THERAPIES

96. How do I find out what clinical trials are available?

Most patients receive information about treatment options from their lymphoma physician. However, you can also find out about clinical trials from the National Cancer Institute. Someone at the institute can be contacted at 1-800-422-6237 or on its Web site at http://www.clinicaltrials.gov/. Other Web sites with helpful information are included in the Appendix.

PART SIX

Coping with Lymphoma

Can I continue to work?

Should I join a support group?

If I am dying, how do I cope?

More . . .

97. Can I continue to work?

The ability of someone to continue working after their diagnosis of lymphoma depends on several factors. These include the type of work involved, the schedule and time demands of the treatment, and the side effects of the treatment. There are people who feel very well and have little or no side effects from their treatment, and their overall strength and endurance are not affected. They have their treatment first thing in the morning and are able to go directly to work. Many people feel that work is a fundamental part of their life. Continuing to work can provide a sense of structure, stability, and normalcy. It is also an opportunity for you to interact with your peers. Even if you are able to continue to work, it's a good idea to discuss your diagnosis with your employer because you will need to take time off for medical appointments and treatments. Your employer will be much more understanding if he or she is aware of the reasons for your absence.

Many people, however, feel impaired and may require rest during the day. If you decide to not work, it's a good idea to contact your employer's human resources department, as they can inform you of the steps necessary to ensure that your medical insurance is not interrupted. You may also benefit from talking to a social worker about your eligibility for disability benefits.

98. Should I join a support group?

Support groups, which are available in most communities, may be designed for all cancer patients or for only lymphoma patients. Support groups usually meet monthly, and family members are generally welcome to attend. A support group may also be available specifically for family members.

Your membership attendance in a support group does not necessarily require that you open up to the group, because you may simply prefer to listen. Often it is comforting to hear the stories of how others cope with a similar illness, and you may gain some very helpful insights. If you are unsure whether you will benefit from attendance, try it once or twice, as there is no obligation to continue. Remember, however, that you may also be able to provide much comfort, support, inspiration, and advice to others in the group, especially if you continue to do well. For contact information, ask your physician, nurse, or social worker. The American Cancer Society and the Leukemia and Lymphoma Society have chapter offices throughout the US.

99. If I am dying, how do I cope?

Because coming to terms with one's death is very difficult for most of us, advanced preparations can help. Honesty and openness with loved ones and friends are very important. Honest communication between the medical team and the patient is also very important. Death is a difficult subject for most of us to discuss, and this is certainly true of most physicians, even oncology and hematology physicians. Too frequently, this subject will not be adequately discussed, sometimes resulting in a sense of mistrust and suspicion between patients and their family members and physicians. It is very important that up-front discussions be held regarding the appropriateness of further treatment when it is unlikely to provide benefit. Patients may wish to continue treatment, even with little hope of any meaningful response. Having the ability to accept that further treatment is unlikely to be beneficial and may actually be harmful is a great step forward in accepting death. Trust in your physician is essential in reaching this realization.

Even if further treatment is not physically harmful, it can deprive you of meaningful quality of life. Accepting that further treatment is futile can actually be very empowering. It can remove much stress and allow you to dedicate your remaining time to those who are most important to you. You may feel physically much better, as further side effects of treatment are avoided. Talking to a minister or social worker can also be helpful.

Once the decision is made not to pursue further active treatment against the lymphoma, hospice may be appropriate. The hospice movement, in which the emphasis is on quality of life as well as symptom and pain management, rather than the length of life, has evolved greatly over the past 100 years. Most hospice facilities provide support to patients in their own home as much as possible.

Advance planning for serious illness includes an advance directive and a **durable power of attorney**. An **advance directive** is a document that states your preferences for treatments that you will or will not accept if you are in a position in which you are unable to make such a decision. This may be the only way the medical team knows and can honor your wishes. Advance directive forms are available from your healthcare facility. An advance directive may cover such issues as a **do not resuscitate order**, which addresses your wishes concerning resuscitation in the event of heart or lung failure. Because resuscitation usually involves life-support apparatus, your decision about this should be made in advance.

A durable power of attorney or a healthcare proxy allows a specific family member to make decisions about your health care in the event that you are incapacitated. The durable power of attorney also allows an individual to make financial and legal decisions.

Accepting that further treatment is futile can actually be very empowering. It can remove much stress and allow you to dedicate your remaining time to those who are most important to you.

Durable power of attorney

A document allowing another person, usually a close relative, to make financial and medical decisions in the event that you are incapacitated.

Advance directive

A legal document that clarifies a patient's wishes in advance in the event a patient is unable to make decisions at a later time and allows the assignment of an alternative individual to make such decisions.

100. What happens if I have no insurance or insufficient insurance coverage?

Patients without insurance (and sometimes even for those with insurance) must carry a significant financial burden because of their illness. The hospital or clinic will tell you to whom you should speak regarding financial options. Most healthcare facilities will have a financial caseworker or social worker to direct you toward some help. Government programs, disability benefits, or volunteer organizations may provide helpful resources.

The American Cancer Society has a list of useful resources on its Web site (www.cancer.org), which includes information regarding Medicaid and Medicare eligibility, and makes the following recommendations regarding dealings with your insurance company:

- Become familiar with your individual insurance plan and its provisions. If you think that you might need additional insurance, ask your insurance carrier whether it is available.

- Submit claims for all medical expenses even when you are uncertain about your coverage.

- Keep accurate and complete records of claims submitted, pending, and paid.

- Keep copies of all paperwork related to your claims, such as letters of medical necessity, bills, receipts, requests for sick leave, and correspondence with insurance companies.

- Get a caseworker, a hospital financial counselor, or a social worker to help you if your finances are limited. Often, companies or hospitals can work with you to make acceptable payment arrangements if you make them aware of your situation.

Do not resuscitate order

A state whereby aggressive life-saving measures, such as cardiopulmonary resuscitation (CPR), will not be undertaken because they are unlikely to prolong useful life.

COPING WITH LYMPHOMA

- Submit your bills as you receive them. If you become overwhelmed with bills, get help. Contact local support organizations, such as your American Cancer Society or your state's government agencies, for additional assistance.

- Do not allow your medical insurance to expire. Pay premiums in full and on time, as it is often very difficult to get new insurance.

Organizations

The American Cancer Society
American Cancer Society National Home Office
250 Williams NW
Atlanta, GA 30303
Phone: 800-ACS-2345 (800-227-2345)
Website: www.cancer.org

American Society of Clinical Oncology
2318 Mill Rd, Suite 800
Alexandria, VA 22314
Phone: 571-483-1300
Website: www.asco.org

American Society of Hematology
2021 L Street NW, Suite 900
Washington, DC 20036
Phone: 202-776-0544
Fax: 202-776-0545
Website: www.hematology.org

Be The Match
3001 Broadway St NE, Suite 100
Minneapolis, MN 55413-1753
Phone: 1-800-MARROW2 (1-800-627-7692)
website: www.bethematch.org

Blood and Marrow Transplant Information Network
2310 Skokie Valley Road, Suite 104
Highland Park, IL 60035
Phone: 888-597-7674
Website: www.bmtinfonet.org

The Bone Marrow Foundation
515 Madison Ave, Suite 1130
New York, NY 10022
Phone: 212-838-3029
Fax: 212-223-0081
Website: www.bonemarrow.org

Cancer Care, Inc.
275 7th Avenue
New York, NY 10001
Phone: 800-813-HOPE (4673)
Website: www.cancercare.org

Cancer Research Institute (CRI)
One Exchange Plaza
55 Broadway, Suite 1802
New York, NY 10006
Phone: 212-688-7515
Fax: 212-832-9376
Website: www.cancerresearch.org

The Center for International Bone and Marrow Transplant Research
The Medical College of Wisconsin Clinical Cancer Center
9200 W. Wisconsin Ave
Suite C5500
Milwaukee, WI 53226
Phone: 414-805-0700
Website: www.cibmtr.org

Department of Veterans Affairs
Veterans Health Association
810 Vermont Avenue, NW
Washington, DC 20420
Phone: 1-877-222-VETS (8387)
Website: www.va.gov

Leukemia & Lymphoma Society of America
National Office
1311 Mamaroneck Ave, Suite 310
White Plains, NY 10605
Phone: 800-955-4572 or 914-949-5213
Fax: 914-949-6691
Website: www.lls.org

Lymphoma Research Foundation
115 Broadway, Suite 1301
New York, NY 10016
Phone: 212-349-2910
or 800-500-9976
Website: www.lymphoma.org

National Cancer Institute
9609 Medical Center Dr.
Bethesda, MD 20892-9760
1-800-4-CANCER (1-800-422-6237)
Website: www.nci.nih.gov
For clinical trial information: www.nci.nih.gov/clinical_trials

National Center for Complementary and Alternative Medicine
9000 Rockville Pike
Bethesda, MD 20898
Phone: 888-644-6226
Website:nccam.nih.gov

National Coalition for Cancer Survivorship
1010 Wayne Avenue, Suite 315
Silver Spring, MD 20910
Phone: 877-NCCS-YES (877-622-7937)
Website: www.canceradvocacy.org

National Comprehensive Cancer Network
275 Commerce Dr., Suite 300
Port Washington, PA 19034
Phone: 888-909-NCCN (888-909-6226) or 215-690-0300
Fax: 215-690-0280
Website: www.nccn.org

Oncology Nursing Society
125 Enterprise Dr.
Pittsburgh, PA 15275
Phone: 866-257-4ONS (866-257-4667)
Fax: 412-859-6162
Website: www.ons.org

Social Security Administration
Office of Public Inquiries
6401 Security Boulevard
Baltimore, MD 21235
Phone: 800-772-1213 or 800-325-0778 (TTY)
Website: www.ssa.gov

Well Spouse Foundation
63 West Main St., Suite H
Freehold, NJ 07728
Phone: 800-838-0879 or 212-685-8815
Website: www.wellspouse.org

Additional Websites with Lymphoma Information

Association of Cancer Online Resources
www.acor.org

Cancer.Net
www.cancer.net

Lymphoma Information Network
www.lymphomainfo.net

Other Websites of Interest

www.aicr.org
The American Institute for Cancer Research
This site discusses methods to reduce the risk of cancer.

www.cancersupportivecare.com/pharmacy.html
This site covers chemotherapy drugs and ways of coping with
their side effects. It also has links to the financial assistance programs of pharmaceutical companies.

www.cms.hhs.gov
This is the website for the Centers for Medicare and Medicaid
Services.

www.dol.gov
Information on the Family and Medical Leave Act can be
found here.

www.needymeds.com
This is an information site for patient financial assistance programs for medications.

www.usda.gov/cnpp/
The U.S. Department of Agriculture; Center for Nutrition Policy
and Promotion. This website focuses on healthy eating habits.

A

Acquired immunodeficiency syndrome (AIDS): The syndrome resulting from infection with the human immunodeficiency virus (HIV).

Acute lymphoblastic leukemia: A fast-growing type of leukemia.

Advance directive: A legal document that clarifies a patient's wishes in advance in the event a patient is unable to make decisions at a later time and allows the assignment of an alternative individual to make such decisions.

Albumin: A special type of protein found in the bloodstream.

Alkylating agents: A class of chemotherapy drugs.

Allogeneic transplant: A transplant using another individual as the donor.

Alopecia: Hair loss.

Alternative therapy: A therapy other than a conventionally accepted medical treatment.

Anemia: A condition marked by a low hemoglobin level.

Anemia of chronic disease: Anemia caused by the bone marrow's reaction to being sick.

Ann Arbor Staging System: Used to describe the areas in the body affected by the lymphoma. It was created at a conference held in Ann Arbor, Michigan.

Anorexia: Loss of appetite.

Antibodies: Specialized proteins of the immune system that help fight infections. They can also be created to recognize proteins on cancer cells, as in some types of lymphoma treatments.

Antibody therapy: The use of antibodies to treat cancer.

Antiemetic: A medication to prevent nausea and vomiting.

Antigen: Any substance that can induce an immune response. Antigens include infections or cancer cells.

Antitumor antibiotics: A class of chemotherapy drugs.

Aorta: The main blood vessel (artery) that carries blood from the heart to the smaller arteries, thereby delivering blood to all parts of the body.

Apheresis catheter: A large indwelling catheter placed through the skin into a large vein to allow the collection of stem cells.

Aplasia: A condition where blood cells are not produced.

Apoptosis: A process by which normal cells die. Some cancer cells do not die, and a failure of cells to undergo apoptosis can contribute to the growth of cancer. It is often referred to as "programmed cell death."

Arteries: The vessels that carry blood cells containing oxygen to the organs and tissues of the body.

Autoimmune disease: An illness in which a person's own immune system mistakenly begins to see certain parts of its own body as foreign, resulting in immunologically driven inflammatory damage to the tissues affected

Autologous stem cell transplant : A transplant in which one is one's own bone marrow stem cell donor.

B

B cell: A type of lymphocyte.

B symptoms: Fevers, night sweats, and weight loss that may occur in lymphoma patients. They can occur individually or together.

Bacteria: One class of infectious agents.

BCNU pneumonitis: Inflammation of the lungs caused by the chemotherapy drug BCNU.

Benign: Not cancerous.

Biologic therapy: Treatment that focuses the body's immune system on diseased cells.

Biopsy: The removal of tissue or a fluid sample for microscopic examination.

Bolus: A rapid intravenous injection.

Bone marrow: Soft substance inside many bones in the body where the blood cells are produced.

Broviac catheter: A type of catheter that goes directly into a large vein to allow easier administration of medications and blood tests.

Burkitt lymphoma: A very rapidly growing and aggressive type of lymphoma.

C

CD20: A protein on the surface of B-lymphocytes and most B-cell lymphomas.

Cellular immune response: The part of the immune response that uses lymphocytes to directly remove antigens. In contrast, the humoral immune response uses antibodies to remove antigens.

Central nervous system (CNS): The brain and spinal cord.

Chemotherapy: Drugs used to treat a disease; the different types of drugs used to treat cancer.

Chronic lymphocytic leukemia (CLL): The most common slow-growing type of leukemia.

Clinical trials: Research studies evaluating promising new treatments in patients.

CNOP: A combination chemotherapy regimen.

Complementary therapy: Therapy used in conjunction with traditional medical treatments.

Complete blood count (CBC): A blood test that takes looks at the red cell count, the hemoglobin, the white count, and the platelet count.

Computed tomography (CT) scan: A specialized type of X-ray that creates a detailed cross-sectional view of the body.

Contrast dye: A chemical that is injected for certain X-rays, including CT scans and MRI scans, that results in better contrast pictures.

Cyclophosphamide, doxorubicin, vincristine, and prednisone: Four drugs that are commonly used together to treat lymphoma.

Cytokines: Chemicals produced by T lymphocytes in order to generate an immune response.

Cytoplasm: The fluid part of a cell that surrounds the central nucleus.

D

Dehydration: Low fluids in the body, which can cause dizziness, fatigue, fainting, and other minor symptoms. If not corrected, dehydration can cause more serious problems.

Depression: A disorder characterized by excessive sadness and feelings of hopelessness.

Deoxyribonucleic acid (DNA): The material that carries the genetic code for each organism or person.

Diaphragm: The large muscle that separates the lungs from the abdomen. Its movement is important for breathing.

Diffuse large B-cell Lymphoma (DLBCL): A type of intermediate-grade lymphoma.

Dimples of Venus: The dimples seen on the skin over the sacrum on the lower back.

Do not resuscitate order: A state whereby aggressive life-saving measures, such as cardiopulmonary resuscitation (CPR), will not be undertaken because they are unlikely to prolong useful life.

Durable power of attorney: A document allowing another person, usually a close relative, to make financial and medical decisions in the event that you are incapacitated.

E

Endoscopy: A procedure to examine the gut with a fiber optic light.

Enzymes: Chemical messengers within the body.

Eosinophils: One type of white blood cell.

Epstein-Barr virus (EBV): The virus that causes infectious mononucleosis and can cause lymphocytes to grow abnormally.

Erythropoietin: A hormone produced by the kidneys that stimulates the bone marrow to produce red blood cells.

Esophagitis: Inflammation of the esophagus.

Esophagus: The tube connecting the throat to the stomach.

F

Fatigue: Tiredness, particularly the debilitating, continuous tiredness that signals illness or disease.

Femur: The thigh bone.

Fibrosis: The replacement of normal tissue with scar tissue.

Fine needle aspiration (FNA): A procedure to obtain a sample of tissue using a small needle.

Flow cytometry: A procedure for examining the proteins present on the surface of cells.

Follicles: Round structures containing lymphocytes.

Follicular Lymphoma International Prognostic Index (FLIPI): A modified form of the IPI for determining the prognosis of patients with follicular lymphomas.

Follicular lymphomas: Lymphomas composed of lymphocytes organized into round structures.

G

Gallium scan: A nuclear medicine test that uses gallium to show areas of lymphoma within the body.

Gastrointestinal tract: The gut, from mouth to anus.

Graft-versus-host disease (GVHD): An illness caused by the donor's immune system recognizing and attacking tissues and organs of the patient.

Graft-versus-lymphoma (GVL): A situation in which the donor's immune system recognizes the recipient's lymphoma cells as foreign and works to eliminate the lymphoma.

Granules: Small particles inside white blood cells that contain enzymes.

Growth factors: Chemicals that can be injected to stimulate the production of blood cells.

H

Hashimoto's thyroiditis: A type of inflammation of the thyroid due to abnormal recognition of the thyroid gland as foreign.

Hematocrit: A measure of the number of red cells, useful for anemia or polycythemia (too many red cells).

Hematology: The study of diseases of the blood, including blood cancers.

Hematopoietic stem cell: The most immature cell that has the capacity to develop into/generate red cells, white blood cells, and platelets throughout a person's life.

Hematologist/oncologist: A physician specializing in the treatment of blood disorders and cancer.

Hemoglobin: A protein present in red blood cells that carries oxygen.

Hepatitis C virus: One of the viruses that can infect the liver and cause chronic liver inflammation.

Hickman catheter: An intravenous line that passes through the skin into a large vein near the heart. It provides a safer and easier way to administer chemotherapy and obtain blood samples.

Hodgkin lymphoma: A type of lymphoma.

Human immunodeficiency virus (HIV): A virus that attacks the human immune system, leaving the carrier prone to infections.

Human leukocyte antigen (HLA) typing: Testing of the transplantation antigens to determine whether two people are compatible for transplantation.

Human T-cell lymphotropic virus type 1 (HTLV-1): A virus that can cause leukemia by infecting T lymphocytes.

Humerus: The major bone connecting the shoulder to the elbow.

Humoral immune response: An immune response that uses antibodies rather than cells to destroy an antigen (foreign protein).

Hyperviscosity: A condition in which the blood is too thick.

I

Idiotype: A protein sequence on the surface of B-lymphocytes that is like a fingerprint. All related lymphocytes contain the same protein sequence.

Immune system: The complex system by which the body protects itself from harmful outside invaders.

Immunoglobulin M (IgM): One of the five different types of antibodies that are part of the immune system.

Immunotherapy: Treatment aimed at controlling the immune system.

Indwelling catheter: An intravenous catheter that can remain in place for longer than a few days.

Indolent: Slow growing.

Indolent lymphomas: A group of lymphomas that are generally slow growing and are usually treated only if causing important symptoms or signs of organ damage.

Infectious mononucleosis: A viral infection caused by the Epstein-Barr virus. Also called glandular fever.

Inferior vena cava: The large vein that carries blood back toward the heart.

Institutional review board (IRB): A group that reviews research studies to ensure they are safe and ethical.

Interferon therapy: A type of immune therapy.

International Prognostic Index (IPI): A system to determine the prognosis of patients with lymphoma.

Interventional radiologist: A physician who is trained in using X-rays to aid in the performance of some types of surgical procedures.

Intramuscular: An injection into the muscle.

Intrathecal: The administration of a substance, often chemotherapy, into the fluid surrounding the spinal cord and brain.

Intravenous immunoglobulin (IVIG): A collection of pooled immunoglobulin G, obtained from many donors.

K

Karnofsky Performance Status scale: A system to evaluate how patients do when performing normal daily activities.

L

Lactate dehydrogenase (LDH): An enzyme measured using a simple blood test.

Laparotomy: Surgery involving an incision to look directly into the abdomen.

Leukapheresis: A procedure to remove large numbers of white blood cells from the body.

Leukopenia: A low white blood cell count.

Libido: Sex drive.

Local treatment: Treatment aimed at a particular area of the body. For example, radiation treatment is local, whereas chemotherapy is systemic.

Low microbial diet: A diet that that limits your exposure to food-borne bacteria or fungi.

Lymphadenopathy: Enlarged lymph nodes.

Lymphangiogram: An X-ray study of lymph glands after they are injected with a dye.

Lymphoblastic lymphoma: An aggressive, fast-growing type of lymphoma.

Lymph fluid: The fluid that carries lymphocytes around the body.

Lymph node architecture: The structure of lymph nodes when they are seen under a microscope.

Lymphocytes: The main type of cell that makes up the immune system. It is the abnormal cell in lymphoma.

Lymphocyte-depleted Hodgkin lymphoma: Another type of Hodgkin lymphoma.

Lymphocyte-rich Hodgkin lymphoma: A type of Hodgkin lymphoma.

Lymphoplasmacytic lymphoma (LPL): The lymphoma associated with Waldenstrom's macroglobulinemia.

Lymphokines: Chemicals that are produced by lymphocytes and help in coordinating the immune response.

Lymphoma: Cancer of the lymphocytes.

Lymphoma classification: A system to organize the many different types of lymphoma.

Lymphatic channels: The tiny vessels that connect the lymph glands.

Lymph glands: The large collections of lymphocytes that exist at intervals throughout the lymph system. They can get big and painful in response to an infection.

Lymph nodes: Another term for lymph glands.

M

Magnetic resonance imaging (MRI): A technique based on the use of magnetic fields to produce images of body parts.

Malaria: An infection caused by a parasite that is transmitted by mosquitoes.

Malignant: Cancerous.

MALT lymphomas: A type of lymphoma that tends to involve lymph glands present in the mucosa (the lining of the gut or other organs).

Marginal zone lymphoma: A type of indolent lymphoma.

Mantle cell lymphoma: An uncommon type of aggressive lymphoma.

Mediastinal nodes: Lymph nodes present in the area between the lungs.

Megakaryocytes: The bone marrow cells that produce platelets.

Megestrol acetate: A medication that can increase the appetite.

Mesenteric lymph nodes: The lymph nodes present in the abdomen tissue that anchors the bowel.

Microtubules: Structures present in individual cells that are important for allowing cells to divide.

Mixed cellularity Hodgkin lymphoma: One of the types of Hodgkin lymphoma.

Monoclonal antibodies: Antibodies that bind to a specific target on the surface of lymphoma or other cancer cells.

Monocytes: One type of white blood cell.

Mucositis: Inflamation of any of the mucous membranes lining the digestive tract from the mouth, down to the esophogus, to the anus.

Mycosis fungoides: A type of lymphoma that mainly involves the skin.

N

Neutropenia: A low level of neutrophils.

Neutrophil: The main type of white blood cell. It is especially important for fighting bacterial infections.

Non-Hodgkin lymphoma: The most common type of lymphoma.

Nonmyeloablative or reduced intensity allogeneic stem cell transplants: A transplant in which the doses of chemotherapy or radiotherapy are reduced compared to those given for a standard transplant.

Nuclear medicine: The medicine specialty that deals with using radioisotopes for obtaining body scans and for treatment.

Nucleoside analogues: A type of chemotherapy drug that targets lymphocytes.

Nucleus: The central part of the cell. It contains the genetic information for that cell.

O

Oncology: The field of medicine that studies cancer.

P

Palpitations: The sensation of an irregular heartbeat.

Pathologist: A physician who makes the diagnosis of lymphoma and other cancers from evaluating biopsies and other surgical specimens under the microscope.

Performance status: The level of ability with which patients can perform their routine daily activities.

Peripheral blood stem cell transplant: A transplant using marrow stem cells that have been obtained from the blood circulation.

Peripheral neuropathy: A condition caused by damage to the nerves in the arms or legs.

Petechiae: Pinpoint red spots that occur with low platelet counts and are due to tiny areas of bleeding into the skin.

Phagocyte: A cell that scavenges other cells.

Phototherapy: A type of therapy using ultraviolet light.

Plasmablastic lymphoma: A rare type of lymphoma due to immature plasma cells.

Plasma cells: The most mature type of B cell. They produce immunoglobulins and are the malignant cells present in multiple myeloma.

Plasmapheresis: A treatment that consists of removing plasma.

Platelets: Tiny blood cells that are produced in the bone marrow and are important for blood clotting.

Pneumocystis jarovecii pneumoniae: An infection affecting the lungs that can occur in people with an abnormal immune system.

Portacath: An indwelling intravenous catheter that is placed entirely underneath the skin.

Positron emission tomography (PET) scan: X-ray studies that use the abnormal sugar metabolism of cancer cells to identify metastatic deposits.

Prognosis: A prediction of the course that a disease will take.

Pulmonary function tests: A set of tests performed to evaluate the ability of the lungs to function properly.

Purging: The technique whereby certain cells (usually cancerous) are removed from the remaining cells present in the collected bone marrow or stem cells.

R

Radiation therapy: Treatment using radiation.

Raynaud's syndrome: A disorder associated with pain and a change in blood flow and color in the fingers.

Red blood cells: The most common type of blood cells that carry oxygen around the body. They carry oxygen to the tissues of the body and help eliminate carbon dioxide from the body by carrying it back to the lungs for elimination.

Reproductive system: The body parts associated with reproduction.

Retroperitoneal lymph nodes: The most common lymph nodes present in the abdomen.

Revised European-American Classification (REAL): The basis of the newest lymphoma classification.

Rheumatoid arthritis: An auto-immune disorder associated with destruction and deformity of joints.

S

Saliva: The lubricating substance produced by the salivary glands that is essential for chewing and swallowing.

Salivary glands: The gland that produces saliva.

Shingles: A painful condition with a rash, usually affecting one area of the skin in the distribution of a nerve. It is due to reactivation of the chickenpox virus and usually occurs when the immune system is depressed.

Simulation: The planning necessary before administering any radiation treatment.

Sjögren's syndrome: An autoimmune disorder causing inflammation of the salivary and lacrimal (tear) glands, resulting in dry eyes and a dry mouth.

Small lymphocytic lymphoma (SLL): A type of indolent lymphoma that is similar to chronic lymphocytic leukemia.

Spinal tap: The procedure for obtaining a sample of spinal fluid.

Spinal fluid: The fluid surrounding the brain and spinal fluid.

Spleen: The large lymph node–like organ under the lower left ribs.

Sporadic Burkitt: The form of Burkitt lymphoma that occurs in the United States.

Stage: A reference to the number of places in the body affected by lymphoma or other cancer.

Stem cell mobilization: The process by which bone marrow stem cells are stimulated to move into blood circulation.

Stem cells: A type of cell that can produce red cells, white cells, and platelets.

Stem cell transplantation: The procedure of replacing bone marrow stem cells to allow recovery of blood cells after high-dose chemotherapy.

Subcutaneous: Underneath the skin.

Superior vena cava syndrome: A condition in which the blood flow back to the heart is decreased due to obstruction, usually by very large lymph nodes.

Systemic lupus erythematosus: A disease in which the immune system attacks the body, causing inflammatory damage to multiple organs, including the skin, kidneys, heart, or brain.

Systemic treatment: A treatment, such as chemotherapy, that reaches all body parts through the bloodstream.

T

T cell: One of the major types of lymphocytes.

Testosterone: A male hormone.

Thrombocytopenia: A low platelet count.

Thymus: An organ behind the breastbone that is important for the development of an immune response, especially in children.

Tissues: A collection of cells of a similar type with a similar function.

Tonsils: Large lymph nodes present in the back of the throat.

Total body irradiation: Radiation therapy administered to the entire body, usually in preparation for a transplant.

Trachea: The windpipe.

Translocation: An abnormality of certain chromosomes seen in some cancer cells.

V

Vaccine: An injection given to stimulate an immune response.

Veins: Blood vessels that return blood to the heart.

Vinca alkaloids: A type of chemotherapy drug.

Viruses: Tiny infectious agents that require other cells for their growth and survival.

W

Waldenstrom's macroglobulinemia (WM): A type of lymphoma that produces too much IgM and can be associated with an increased viscosity.

White blood cells: Blood cells that are most important for fighting infection.

Working formulation: One of the lymphoma classifications.

X

Xerostomia: Dryness of the mouth due to disease.

Note: Page numbers followed by *f* or *t* indicate material in figures or tables respectively.

A

INDEX

prognosis, 38
prognostic model, 106
progressive multifocal
    leukoencephalopathy (PML), 116
proteasomes, 170
PTLD. *See* post transplant
    lymphoproliferative disorders
pulmonary function tests, 99
purging, 189

R

R-CODOX-M/IVAC, 123
R-EPOCH, 123
R-ESHAP, 124
R-ICE, 124
radiation port, 160
radiation therapy, 44, 89, 117, 159–160
    side effects of, 161–163
    treatment of, 160–161
radioimmunotherapy agents, 114
radioimmunotherapeutic antibodies, 167
Rai staging system, 51
Raynaud's syndrome, 55
re-biopsy, 45
REAL. *See* Revised European-
    American Lymphoma
    Classification
rectal examinations, 96
red blood cells, 4, 5, 12
reduced intensity conditioning (RIC),
    186–187
reproductive system, 145
retroperitoneal lymph nodes, 40
Revised European-American Lymphoma
    Classification (REAL), 32
rheumatoid arthritis, 4
rheumatologic abnormalities, 81
RIC. *See* reduced intensity
    conditioning
rituximab, 114, 120, 167, 168
romadepsin, 170–171

S

saliva, 29, 162
salivary glands, 63
salvage chemotherapy, 131
SCID. *See* severe combined
    immunodeficiency
secondary cutaneous lymphoma, 86
serious illness, advance planning for, 202
serum lactate dehydrogenase, 101
serum viscosity, 55
severe combined immunodeficiency
    (SCID), 76
sexuality, treatment affecting, 155–156
Sezary syndrome, 87, 88
shingles, 139
simulation, 159
Sjögren's syndrome, 28–29, 63
skin, 86–87
small lymphocytic lymphoma (SLL),
    50–53
"snapshot" probabilities, 100
spinal cord compression, 161
spinal tap, 126
spleen, 2, 3, 6
splenic marginal zone lymphoma, 62
sporadic Burkitt lymphoma, 72–73
staging laparotomy, 127–128
staging of Lymphoma, 37–42, 37*t*
standard uptake value (SUV), 43
Stanford V regimen, 129
stem cell mobilization, 177
stem cell transplant, 79, 171–173
stem cells, 7, 181
subcutaneous, 86, 134
superior vena cava syndrome, 20
support groups, 200–201
SUV. *See* standard uptake value
syngeneic transplant, 181
systemic lupus erythematosus, 4, 29
systemic treatment, 134